THE UNMEDICAL BOOK

How to Conquer Disease,
Lose Weight, Avoid Suffering
& Save Money

by

Elizabeth and Dr. Elton Baker

D1569937

THE UNMEDICAL BOOK

How to Conquer Disease, Lose Weight, Avoid Suffering & Save Money

by

Elizabeth and Dr. Elton Baker

Drelwood Publications

Distributed by

COMMUNICATION CREATIVITY
Box 213
Saguache, CO 81149

The information in this book is presented as a matter of general interest only and not as prescribing cures. Readers must use their own judgment, consult a holistic medical expert or their personal physician for specific applications to their individual problems. The authors and publisher assume no responsibility for errors, inaccuracies, omissions or any inconsistency herein.

The following trademarks appear in this book: Band-Aid, Chloromycetin, Coumadin, Elavil, NutraSweet, Novocain, Thiuretic, Ser-Ap-Es, Dicumarol, Wasa.

Library of Congress Cataloging-in-Publication Data

Baker, Elizabeth,
 The UNmedical Book

 Bibliography: p.
 Includes index.
 1. Naturopathy—popular works. 2. Nutrition.
3. Raw food diet. 4. Reducing. I. Baker, Elton,
II. Title.
RZ440.B28   1987   615.5'35   87–6775
ISBN 0–918880–14–9

Printed and bound in the United States of America

ALSO AVAILABLE FROM
CATHERINE COWLES

The Tattered & Torn Series
Tattered Stars
Falling Embers
Hidden Waters
Shattered Sea
Fractured Sky

Sparrow Falls
Fragile Sanctuary
Delicate Escape
Broken Harbor
Beautiful Exile
Chasing Shelter
Secret Haven

The Lost & Found Series
Whispers of You
Echoes of You
Glimmers of You
Shadows of You
Ashes of You

The Wrecked Series
Reckless Memories
Perfect Wreckage
Wrecked Palace
Reckless Refuge
Beneath the Wreckage

The Sutter Lake Series
Beautifully Broken Pieces
Beautifully Broken Life
Beautifully Broken Spirit
Beautifully Broken Control
Beautifully Broken Redemption

Standalone Novels
Further to Fall
All the Missing Pieces

For a full list of up-to-date Catherine Cowles titles,
please visit catherinecowles.com.

Dedication

We dedicate this book to four nutritional physicians who stand tall in their work and commitment to listening to and treating the whole person, their patient. The first is Lloyd Silver, M.D., whose faith in God, knowledge and experience helped us start on the long road back to health; to Joseph Morgan, M.D., in whose fasting clinic we discovered all our allergies, the causes of most of our illnesses; to Jonathan Collin, M. D., whose vast knowledge of nutrition and whose interest in continued learning is an inspiration as well as a help. Lastly to the memory of William A. Ellis, D. O., eminent practitioner of nutritional medicine for over forty years, lecturer and teacher of nutrition to doctors and to audiences on radio and television for ten years.

Acknowledgments

To write a list of all those accommodating librarians and wonderful people in the United States of America, Europe and Australia to whom we owe so much in compiling information for this book would be next to impossible. For the help of many professionals and for the countless bits of valuable information from the experiences of family, friends and acquaintances that have gone into the fabric of the text, we wish to express deepest appreciation.

Our loving thanks go to our children and grandchildren for giving us moral support. We are especially grateful for the patience and the endurance demonstrated by our faithful editors, Tom and Marilyn Ross, as we all labored, sometimes behind schedule, on the manuscript.

May God bless you, one and all.

Table of Contents

Foreword 11

Preface 13

PART I.   What It's All About:
            Nutrition for Radiant Health 15

PART II.   An Encyclopedia of Natural Therapies
            to Help Conquer Problems and
            Diseases 23

PART III.   Healthy Weight Control:
            An Actual Class History 167

PART IV.   Our Personal Stories 203
            Elizabeth Triumphs Over Cancer
            Elton Masters Glaucoma

PART V.   Appendix 213
            Why a Vegetarian Diet?
            The Advantages of Organically Grown Food
            The Merits of Health Food Stores
            High, Medium and Low Energy Foods
            Supplements: To Take of Not to Take?
            The Beauties of Wheat Grass
            Deadly Don'ts
            Body pH Chart
            Kinesiology Testing for Adults
            Children's Kinesiology Testing
            Hypoglycemia Symptoms
            Exercises of the Astronauts
            Measurement/Equivalent Tables

PART VI. Directory of Products,
Sources & Services 237

Glossary 241

Bibliography 253

Index 257

Order Form 265

Foreword

I've been motivated to share the principles behind my own 30 years of experience in using an alternative nutritional program to conquer disorders and diseases with a few select patients. One of these was Letha (Elizabeth) Baker. She has applied the same principles to her own health problems and, with the cooperation of her husband, Elton, has been prompted in turn to further pursue the subject of wholistic/natural healing.

From their own experiences, and by careful observation of the course of others whom they were able to help, a wealth of natural preventive and therapeutic information accumulated. It has been alphabetically organized for the convenience of the reader seeking help to live a natural alternative lifestyle. This, their third book, is an excellent companion to their first work, *The UNcook Book.*

I highly recommend the Baker's *UNmedical Book* as a guide to boost the immune system and thus, as an effective way to prevent the rampant onslaught of disease. Additionally, it is a guide to the treatment of many disabling and life-threatening maladies of our modern society. These maladies are largely due to increasing dependence on scientific knowledge in the medical and environmental fields.

Lloyd H. Silver, M.D.

Preface

It is as nutrition researchers, teachers and writers trying to use nature's way that we make known what we observe, learn and experience. The recommendations we make are not meant to be prescriptive, but can be used as flexible programs when working with your doctor. No book can substitute for competent professional care.

We wish to state that in all cases of serious illness, people should see a licensed physician for a diagnosis of the problem or problems. Then by making their own decisions for the kind of treatment or therapy they wish to accept, and taking the responsibility for their own health, individuals can exert their power of choice. They can choose to go the orthodox medical way of treatment—or they can choose natural, nutritional, drugless therapies.

We are reporters. We are experimenters. We choose to trust God and the natural ways He taught. They did not fail us. God's word, as recorded in the Bible, is the source of information upon which we built this book of natural, low-cost therapies and optimum nutrition. God told man how to maintain a healthy body; how to live, think, and eat for it to heal in case of accident or illness.

Our book may be considered experimental. But it is verified by successful case histories of many individuals over considerable time. We do not claim any of the modalities mentioned in this book are cures. Only the body cures itself, given the necessary substance for repair and maintenance. This is one of the great truths. May you, our precious reader, receive the blessings of experiencing this truth.

Elizabeth Baker, M.A.
Elton Baker, M.S., Ph.D.

Part I

What It's All About: Nutrition for Radiant Health

From the expressed need of our audiences came the inspiration and the burden on our hearts to write this book. Wherever we appear on television and radio or lecture, from Australia to Amsterdam and across the length and breadth of the United States, people eagerly seek ways they can effectively cope with the responsibility of their own health. They ask what *they* themselves can do about it. In this book we try to answer that question. We discuss many problems and diseases that we, our family, friends and acquaintances have overcome, prevented or improved. Whole foods, natural supplements, exercising and faith are the tools to good health. They are augmented with dedication, persistence, thanksgiving and by following God's ways.

We pray each person can find a nutrition oriented M.D., naturopath, osteopath, homeopath or chiropractor and dentist for help when needed. These caring, people-oriented professionals listen to their patients, encourage and guide them in self help. They treat them as individuals, never overlooking the fact no two are alike. They are called alternate therapists by many. Their therapies and treatments are referred to as alternate or nontoxic therapies. With tongue in cheek, they call themselves the medical underground because their practice does not always follow the powerful dictates of the American Medical Association (AMA). They use sparingly the cut (surgery), burn (radiation and x-ray), and poison (drug) methods of conventional medicine. Their natural ways of treating help people get well. They help the body to "cure" itself. (We dare to use this word that medical orthodoxy avoids. Perhaps it's because in their practice they rarely see cure. These unorthodox physicians mainly see improvement in those they treat and guide.)

Let us give a couple of examples. All through the 1960's and early 1970's Elizabeth suffered dozens of distressing symptoms. She had headaches, digestive malfunction, constipation, fatigue that led to almost constant exhaustion, irritability, restless achy legs, intense hunger, nausea, hot sweats, bursitis, Raynaud's syndrome, poor memory, tinnitus (noises in the ears), diarrhea, and numbness in hands and feet. Through those years she consulted no less than twenty-one doctors. She went through four clinics, and was hospitalized a total of eight times at a cost of more than $150,000. Test after test revealed nothing drastically wrong. She was ultimately labeled a mental case and sent to psychiatrists. After reading *Body, Mind and Sugar* by E.M. Abrahamson and A.W. Peget, she suspected hypoglycemia (low blood sugar).

After reading *Low Blood Sugar and You* by Carlton Frederick, she knew it was hypoglycemia for she had all but one of the many symptoms he mentioned. After this, her great "discovery," she could get no doctor to even listen to her, much less help her. One said he knew hypoglycemia was fashionable among women. Another called it a fad. Several advised her to eat something like a milkshake or candy bar for quick energy (the worst possible thing). A few admitted they knew nothing about hypoglycemia. One hospital-clinic flatly stated there was no such thing as hypoglycemia. (In the 1970's they finally had to come around to the fact hypoglycemia did exist, but chose to call it hyperinsulinism, which of course is just as accurate a terminology.)

Elizabeth finally found a doctor who would write out the order for a six-hour glucose tolerance test. When it came time to report the results, he had his nurse call. She gushed, "You have hypoglycemia. You *really* do." She relayed several questions to the doctor who answered them briefly from the background. When Elizabeth asked to talk to him, he refused to come to the phone.

Since that time we have listened to hundreds of people whose tragic story of poor health and constant fatigue closely resembled Elizabeth's. Many physicians say some fifty percent of the population suffers from low blood sugar. Thank heaven, a much larger percentage of orthodox physicians now know what to do about it.

To get over hypoglycemia Elizabeth had to get off all sugar, white flour products, white rice and processed foods. (Most of them have sugar.) Through diagnostic fasting (see APPEN-DIX, Diagnostic Fasting) she determined what foods she was allergic to, then eliminated them completely. Her severest allergies, as with most people, were sugar and wheat. Allergists say at least ninety percent of Americans are allergic to sugar and at least sixty percent to wheat. We don't quite agree with this. From our seventeen years of experience researching nutrition, writing, lecturing and teaching, we would move both percentages up!

Now, years later and still on an all raw diet, Elizabeth is free of hypoglycemia and degenerative disease. At seventy-three, that is pretty terrific.

Elton also recovered, through natural therapies, from a degenerative disease, oftentimes spoken of as "incurable" by orthodox physicians. All his adult life he had suffered from asthma. One attack was so severe he was hospitalized for days with what doctors at first thought was a heart attack. All through the 1960's, he wheezed every night after dinner. Three different doctors told him the stress of teaching college along with managing a business of thirty-five employees was the cause. One physician said he was no doubt resenting having to overwork to put two sons through college and "live with an ailing wife."

Then Elizabeth quit sugar. The day after, she had no pain in her arthritic hands and elbows. In a few days she looked better. Then she got off all wheat and processed foods. Improvement continued. She had Addison's disease and chose to follow Adelle Davis instead of the doctors who said she had perhaps two years to live. Elton was so impressed, he quit sugar too; then a little later wheat, white rice and most processed foods. For the first time in years, he didn't wheeze or have to struggle for breath. A short while before this, he'd undergone his biannual physical examination required by the college. Blood pressure 180/90. Cholesterol 240. Pulse 78. The doctor told him he'd better leave off eggs and eat margarine and cooking oil instead of butter.

But Elton knew the natural kind of cholesterol in eggs was not the kind that did harm. The cholesterol occurring in natural foods is in fine particles that freely goes in and out the cell walls. Every cell of the body needs cholesterol. Whether we get it in our food or not, our bodies are going to synthesize (make) it. The cholesterol particles that our bodies manufacture out of refined carbohydrates, like sugar and white flour, are large and cannot readily go in and out of the cell walls. They get stuck and pile up in the arteries to form obstructive cholesterol deposits that narrow the channels and impede the flow of blood.

When Elton, who is a chemist, studied these facts through, he realized it was wise to take all the bad things out of the diet— processed foods *and the blood pressure pills* that had been prescribed. Another of the processed foods he researched was hydrogenated oil and margarine. Stripped of most of their nutrition in the heat-chemical process, they cannot be digested nor properly expelled by the body. They end up coating the artery walls with sticky plaque. (Cholesterol deposits are on top of sticky plaque.) Naked, nutritionless sugar robs the body of countless nutrients such as vitamins, enzymes and minerals, as the body attempts to utilize it for energy.

With a cleaned up, almost natural diet, and a daily exercise program, Elton began to feel a lot different. He had better energy and stamina. He could think more clearly. He rarely had a cold. His next physical showed the following: blood pressure 138/78; cholesterol 140 (almost one half what it had been); pulse 68. The doctor dismissed him by saying, "The medication has been effective. Keep on taking it yet a little while. Your blood pressure could go back up." Little did he know! He never once asked any questions. There was no opportunity to tell him Elton hadn't taken one dose of the blood pressure medicine, and had changed his diet from a processed one to mainly a natural one. He could have forced that information upon the physician, but a sixth sense suggested it would probably not be listened to because the physician was not familiar with nutrition therapy.

Elton left wondering how he could communicate some of the impressive truths he and Elizabeth had found; truths discovered and rediscovered by eminent, nutrition minded physicians and biochemists across the land whose written words are so grossly under read. From those ponderings was born a newspaper column called *Nutrition News,* which Elton wrote for several years, and in which he retold many of those truths that work so well.

Many patients of alternate therapists *do* get well, *do* mostly stay free of degenerative disease when they follow their therapist/physicians' advice. Through nutrition and natural preventive methods they enjoy a high quality of physical, mental, emotional and spiritual life.

If this is true, you say, then why doesn't every one know about it? For some satanic reason, the mainline press, much of radio and commercial television, the federal government, the Food and Drug Administration (FDA) will not print or communicate those facts. They suppress them. They are threatened by them. After all, if ninety percent of surgery does not need to be done, as the well known M.D. Robert Mendelsohn flatly states in his books and lectures, then at least fifty percent of hospital income would fall off. And most surgeons, anesthesiologists and related staff would be out of jobs. Many internists who diagnose with the aid of X-rays, probing instruments, scanners, etc., would have very few patients; and an army of technicians throughout the medical industry, the second largest industry in the United States of America, would be unemployed.

The foundation of today's conventional medical world is surgery, radiation, X-ray and drugs. Remove even a third of these methods of treatment and the whole structure would begin tumbling down. Is it any wonder these professionals functioning within the established medical world jealously defend the source of their living (their very life blood)? Is it surprising they viciously attack those who help turn sick patients to well people and so eliminate their reason for being?

How many people do you know who are worse off than ever after surgery? Who are still sick after countless visits to doctors, clinics and hospitals? Who have been told we all live with some physical problems? Who conclude from their pathetic search that there is no recovery for them?

Today's orthodox physicians treat symptoms. They study the sick body. They find the problems, locate the trouble spots, then treat them with cut (surgery), burn (radiation), and poison (drug) modalities. Fifty years or so of treating disease instead of treating the patient has proven to be a colossal failure. If you doubt it, read the statistics on the steady increase of most degenerative diseases in the last several decades.

Almost invariably the stories of orthodox treatment are fraught with failure, with disappointment, with weakness and with death. Those of alternate therapies usually have a happy ending. It is incredible to us that so many are still being led astray like sheep, blindly following the doctors whose methods of caring for the sick ignore the only way the body can rejuvinate itself or maintain its vigorous health. Nutrition is what it needs for recovery and restoration. Those doctors wouldn't think of using just a bucket of nails to repair an orginally beautiful but badly abused clinic they wanted to move into. So why do they treat human patients with just drugs and usually no word about nutrition, the best medicine of all?

God intended us to enjoy good health. He told us what to eat in both the first and last books of the Bible. Fruits, all tree and seed bearing fruits, not only apples, peaches, etc., but peas, tomatoes, okra, squash, etc. Genesis 1:29, "And God said, 'Behold, I have given you every herb bearing seed which is upon the face of all the earth, and every tree, in which is the fruit of a tree yielding seed; to you it shall be for meat.'" Revelation 22:2, "...the tree of life which bare twelve manner of fruits and yielding her fruit every month; and the leaves of the tree were for the healing of the nations."

God gave man the teeth of a vegetarian-fruitarian and the digestive system to match. Let us illustrate. Carnivores (meat eating animals) have sharp, pointed teeth for tearing. Vegetarians have cutting, biting and grinding teeth—actually twenty teeth, five on each side below and above, for pulverizing hard foods such as seeds, nuts, grains and fibrous leafy vegetables (the "leaves" of Rev. 22:2). The acid of the carnivore's stomach is extremely strong to break down the flesh proteins he eats. His intestines are short for expelling the meat before it becomes putrefactive. By contrast the stomach acid of humans is less caustic than that of carnivores. Their intestines are three times longer because they need more time for breaking down and digesting the nutrients of fibrous fruits, vegetables, seeds and nuts. When meat, which is a carnivore's diet, is put through the long gut of the vegetarian, it cannot avoid becoming putrefactive.

God told man to eat leaves for the healing. This applies to *all* animals. What do dogs or cats frequently do early in the morning? Eat a bit of green grass or some other green leaf. They instinctively know it is good for them. It is healing. It is medicine. Man, on the other hand, has a problem eating meats. His stomach lacks sufficient acid for proper digestion, and his small intestines and colon are so long the meat becomes rotted before it can be expelled.

After the flood when Noah, his family, and the animals came out of the Ark, God allowed them to eat flesh because there was little other food. But He was careful to instruct them (Leviticus) not to eat pigs, rabbits, webfooted fowl (ducks, geese) and all finless fish, or crustacea (scavengers) because their flesh is unclean. God knew His people would eat flesh raw because they were accustomed to eating everything raw. He did not want them to eat the things that would poison, sicken and kill them.

Before the flood, people were vegetarian. Some lived to be nearly 1,000 years old. Methuselah lived 969 years. After the flood the life span steadily dropped to 100 or fewer years. (The putrefaction in the gut from meat reenters the blood stream through the veins of the intestinal walls. This poison in the blood is the beginning of degenerative disease and the life shortening, aging process.)

It is not a sin to eat flesh. God allows it. The choice is left to us. But let us share another illustration of the way nutrition affects our bodies. When Moses led the children of Israel out of their captivity in Egypt, he provided manna (plant) for them to eat in the wilderness. After several years many of them began complaining about the food, some even wishing they were back in captivity where they could eat the rich, spicy, heavy foods of the Egyptians. It made God angry. Although He had provided the perfect vegetarian food to give them optimal health, vitality, and longevity, they were so ungrateful as to ask for something different. In His infinite love for His children and His permissive will, He indulged them to eat the flesh of a bird, probably grouse, and sent coveys of them in abundance. *Not until they ate this flesh was there sickness and death among His people.*

Statistics show vegetarians live longer than those who eat animal flesh. They are also freer of degenerative disease. The Hunzakuts of the small valley tucked deep into the Himalayas between Pakistan and Russia, eat a mostly vegetarian diet, much of it raw. In late winter when food is scarce they may eat a little meat. Degenerative disease is practically nonexistent. Women eighty look no more than forty and men sometimes procreate at ninety, according to Renee Taylor who lived with the Hunzas for the summer months and wrote an excellent book about it. There is no osteoporosis, no mental retardation, no birth defects. Juvenile delinquency, crime, sexual abnormalities, hate, fear, and jealousy are almost unknown.

There are similar instances of small groups of peoples in isolated areas of the world. Two Indian tribes in the high valleys of the Andes of Bolivia cultivate the rich glacial soil to raise many seed bearing, edible fruits and vegetables. Their consumption of goat and/or llama meat and goat milk is rare. Like the Hunzas, they eat meat only in late winter when other food becomes scarce. Also like the Hunzas, they expect to live to be 100 years old or more. And the Georgians of Southern Russia across the border from Turkey live that long. Their vegetarian diet is complemented with some cultured, unprocessed milk foods along with the dregs of honey that contain highly nutritious traces of bee pollen, propolis and comb. The long living, healthy Bavarians of fifty years ago were lactovegetarians, their unprocessed milk usually cultured and eaten as a yogurt-kefir type of food or as homemade cheese. Until "civilized" man made health cripples of them with sugar and cooked, processed, canned and packaged foods, Eskimos lived relatively disease free lives and went off to die in a lone igloo when they sensed their old bodies should be laid to rest. Their food was mostly fish and whale blubber, all of which they ate raw. This food fare contained the minerals and vitamins, pure and undestroyed by cooking that their sturdy bodies needed to live strong, healthy, long lives.

We all need to return to primitive diets. Therein dwells vigorous health for body, mind and spirit. The choice is ours. Those of us who have made that choice realize these truths with joyous elation. This book is a loving, dedicated attempt to convey an understanding of these truths whose source is the Bible. Our dedication is to help people help themselves to recover or maintain vigorous health. Our prayer is, as many enlightened doctors and related health professionals are teaching their patients, that each functioning adult may take the responsibility for his/her own health.

Part II

An Encyclopedia
of Natural Therapies to Help
Conquer Problems and Diseases

This section contains problems we, our family, and many acquaintances have confronted, and what we did to cope with or solve them. The reader must bear in mind that each person is different. It is the individual with his or her unique set of physical characteristics and problems, his or her mental and emotional condition, that must be studied in a given environment.

We do not advocate or suggest the stated regimen for each specific illness or problem be tried. We only relate to the interested reader what one family and circle of acquaintances did to help themselves after much study, medical advice and scientific counseling.

ABSCESSES (skin): boils, carbuncles, impetigo or other infections of the skin.

There is nothing like balanced nutrition to recover from such skin infections. Healthy, well nourished people do not have them. To cleanse the blood and make up deficiencies that so often accompany these skin eruptions, in addition to an optimal diet of natural foods, such supplements as vitamins A, E, C and D, carrot and beet juice, and zinc have been found to be effective.

For a carbuncle when Elizabeth's body was run down, her nutritionist physician had her take vitamins A, 50,000 IU, E, 600 IU and C, 12,000 milligrams (12 grams), plus beet and carrot juice with leafy green vegetables. She has since learned zinc helps in the healing. The carbuncle was completely gone in three weeks, which most people consider remarkable.

Recently a woman had an old worsening carbuncle on her leg with red streaks extending from it. She decided to try a remedy

Elizabeth had just read about. That was to pack as much white sugar on the infected spot as possible and bind it loosely. It was a joy to treat. The bandage removed easily, it didn't hurt and each morning and night it was "beautifully better." The fifth day after reporting every morning, she called to say the redness and the abscess were completely healed. She was ecstatic. Quite frankly, we were amazed to learn that sugar apparently draws all the moisture, apparently in short order, out of the bacteria and virus cells and so leaves them dead.

ACNE (Acne Vulgaris): an inflammatory disease involving the oil glands and hair follicles of the skin.

Acne plagues several million young people and is increasing rapidly. Studies of it show that this rise is in direct proportion to the decreasing nutrition of the teenage diet.

While there are still those in the professions who say diet has little or nothing to do with acne, many others are quietly going about healing acne by natural nutrition and eliminating those foods the acne patient is allergic or sensitive to. This often turns out to be most of the things a teenager thinks necessary to be happy.

Besides testing for food allergies (see appendix—Kinesiology Testing), and eliminating the offenders, an acne experiencer should avoid all table sugar, products made of white flour, soft drinks, refined foods, artificial sweeteners, chocolate, butter, meat, iodized salt, cheese and homogenized milk. He or she may eat a little bit of sea salt. Dermatologists stress cleanliness of the skin, sunshine at least several minutes almost every day, regular exercise and sufficient sleep. An all-natural diet, possibly with a potassium supplement, should be adhered to.

A fifteen-year-old boy we helped was a year getting off all allergen-causing foods. His acne mostly cleared, returning noticeably when he ate or drank some of the offenders. Disillusioned, this young person had a hair analysis with a coordinating blood analysis. After his physician gave him the results, he went all the way with the diet recommendation. He was out of high school and had a wonderful scholarship for college. It was *his* decision to adopt the all-natural, mostly raw, diet, learning to sprout some seeds for his own needs, and making himself learn to like fresh vegetables. At first he "got them down" with a seasoned to taste yogurt; or almond butter thinned with water; or guacamole, or tehini mixed with mashed garbanzos, lemon juice and dill weed. Fresh fruits were easy to learn to like, as were whole grain breads (in moderation) and crackers. He ate whole grain cornmeal, oats and millet for the first time in his life. His supplements were vitamins A, E, B, C and D; the minerals (all chelated), calcium, magnesium, zinc, and selenium. We recommended chlorophyll as is found in green leafy vegetables and sunshine, both nature's outstanding healers. No-no's were animal fat except for a little raw butter; animal proteins until the acne cleared completely, then chicken, fish and soft cooked eggs once a week.

Two years later a changed young man of twenty-one, in his junior year, bounced by to see us. We hardly knew him with his healthy, smooth, tanned skin and his handsome moustache. He said in spite of many little eating "sins" now and then, his progress was steady, although "painfully" slow, once he began picturing himself free of the stigma of acne. He wrote a little verse: "A body well treated, will have acne deleted." We celebrated by taking him to the restaurant of his choice. Where else but a salad bar?

AGORAPHIBIA: see CLAUSTROPHOBIA

AGING: loss of youth; the process of growing old.

In the mid sixteenth century, countless centuries before de Soto set out for the New World in search of gold and the Fountain of Youth, people avidly sought ways to put off old age. In seeking the magic elixir, the miracle potion, they overlooked the most obvious answer, their diet.

In small areas of the world like Hunzaland in the Himalayas, the high mountain valleys of the Andes, and, a province in Southern Russia, the people live to well over 100 years, are rarely sick physically, mentally or emotionally, and die in their sleep without pain. These people all normally have a diet of primarily raw vegetarian fare.

Our processed, nutrition-deficient, additive-loaded, constipation-causing diet not only invariably heads us into disease, it ages us prematurely. Many of us who have changed to a natural, unprocessed diet have not only gotten over terminal illnesses (in conventional medical parlance) but have reversed some aging processes to the extent that we look younger than the average person our age. To stay young in body and mind the way God planned, we must eat the natural foods He taught us.

Modern medical science has come up with several modalities that are helping thousands slow down the aging process. Live cell therapy as developed by Dr. Niehans of Switzerland over fifty years ago has a rejuvenating effect. Live cells from an embryo calf or lamb organ are injected in the buttock of the patient, are quickly carried by the circulation systems, then deposited in the matching organ. The new live cells act as a booster to the tired cells of the recipient organ and in months can make noticeable improvement. The rich, the famous, movie stars, and politicians have benefited for fifty years from live cell therapy, obtainable until recently only in Europe. At least three clinics in Mexico, two in Tijuana, B.C., and one in Chihuahua, Chili, offer live cell therapy.

Another modality that has proven to be rejuvenating is Gerovital H3, developed by Professor Dr. Ana Aslan in Romania. After developing the formula, she presented it at a world medical congress in the 1950's. Since that time thousands upon thousands from all over the world have gone to Romania for a series of injections or tablets of GH3, as it is called. The formula is mainly a simple one of procaine, which acts like and enhances the action of vitamin B6, and para amino benzoic acid (PABA). Side reactions are rare, advocates claim. It is now available in some states.

Yet another formula, this time developed by an American physician, has rejuvenating properties, especially for scar tissue and as an oxygen enhancer. Called Rodaquin, it is a collection of compounds necessary for all cells to keep renewing themselves with genetic integrity. It works subtly in any or all parts of the body for any ailing organ or diseased area according to both clinical and individual patient reports. The physician who developed it and used it with notable results was so persecuted by orthodox medical establishments he fled to Brazil where the product was held in high esteem by doctors. Although the courts finally ruled in his favor, because of lawsuits and threatened suits, he lived in Brazil until his death. The Rodaquin formula was eventually taken to Mexico where it is made under the exacting and watchful eyes of American medical scientists and technicians.

It is revealing of the state of dictatorial orthodox medicine and collaborating federal government agencies that two outstanding modalities from Europe have been banned for fifty years, and the one developed in the United States by a dedicated, scholarly American doctor is also banned in this country. Many doctors could give patients little hope for all kinds of degenerative diseases, including cancer, until they tried Rodaquin. It is a painless, noninvasive natural preparation that according to reports, gives them not only extended life, but quality health and performance.

AIDS: Acquired Immune Deficiency Syndrome. A disease involving a defect in cell-mediated immunity that has a long incubation period, follows a protracted and debilitating course and is manifested by various opportunistic infections.

In all that has been written or spoken on AIDS since it recently reared its ugly head to frighten the world, a mere token of words have been uttered on the role nutrition could play in combating this dread disease. Yet nutrition is the most important of all considerations. If every bite gives energy, the body can overcome. And every bite *can* give energy.

Soon after the world was made aware of the ominous consequences of AIDS, an experience so greatly impressed us that we feel compelled to relate it. A well educated, accomplished young woman whom we had known since infancy came for a conference. She was a young, beautiful, artistically talented person who had been promiscuous since age fifteen. Her severe symptoms, her nearly unendurable problems, as she reported them in great detail, were those of quite advanced AIDS. We feared she was too ill, too weak and discouraged, to take care of herself. However, she vowed she would follow to the letter any health program we might suggest for her. She had taken a month of sick leave from her management job to recover her health.

We gave her a copy of the program Elizabeth had followed for cancer recovery. It had pulled Elizabeth through in spite of a low immune system, in spite of a weakened body, and a bad digestive system. Then we mentioned Kinesiology Testing for food and environmental allergies and taking vinegar baths (two cups vinegar in a tub of water); and alternate douches of vinegar (two tablespoons per quart of water) and Vitamin C (four grams per quart); strained wheat grass juice (six ounces with two ounces of water); lemon juice (one teaspoon per quart of water). We emphasized days of no stress for this woman, fresh air at all times, stretch exercises and walking as much as energy permitted. We stressed the optimum diet of sprouted seeds,

grains and legumes, fresh raw vegetables and fruits, primary
yeast and spirulina plankton. As she left Elizabeth reminded her
to be on God's side and hold to the faith. This young woman
needed His help. With her soul in her expressive eyes, she
agreed.

For over a year we did not hear of or see her for we were
traveling much of the time. Then one day a mutual friend of
many years told Elizabeth the young woman had been "very,
very ill" but was completely recovered as a result of following
some nutritionists' food intake program. In another year she
was married and the next year had a big, beautiful baby. She now
has a happy healthy family secure in God's love and grace.

From the *Natural Health Magazine of Australia* for October,
1986, comes the story of a young man's recovery from AIDS. In
early 1985, after deteriorating health following severe bronchitis, for which he was given a strong antibiotic, he suffered
dollar-size lumps on neck and groin, herpes, fungal dermatitis,
Kaposi's Sarcoma and extremely low energy. The diagnosis at
the hospital was full blown AIDS with the information that
ninety percent of such cases had a life expectancy of two years or
less. The toxic therapies offered were interferon, chemotherapy
and antiviral drugs (found to be ineffective there). After reading
papers of some American men recovering from AIDS on all-
natural diets, the young man, given the name of a naturopath by
a social worker, chose the nontoxic holistic therapies. The
hospital specialist told him, "They can do no harm, nor can they
do any good."

After following the recommended vegetarian diet, the taking
of fresh, raw vegetable juices and vitamin and mineral supplements, the young man's energy increased, he started playing
squash and tennis again, the lymph nodes were shrinking and
his T4 cell count increased to 250. Then again he had an attack
of bronchitis.

Back in the clinic, he was given a powerful, broad-spectrum
antibiotic. As it turned out, he became so allergic to it his health
rapidly went down. In a month the Kaposi's Sarcoma had
spread throughout his body, the T4 cell count dropped to
ninety-eight, the lymph nodes were larger than before, and the
large patches of fungal dermatitis came back. He was weak,
depressed and frequently confused. He had a blood transfusion,
but refused chemotherapy and cortisone.

Again he consulted a naturopath (his first one had moved

away) who found that he had Candida Albicans, a symptom causing sickening mold-like yeast overgrowth. His holistic therapist prescribed an antifungal drug, a diet that eliminated yeast foods (mainly yeast breads and products, and sugar), mineral and vitamin supplements, vegetable juices, visualization and meditation.

As December 1985 gave way to January, February, and March, he began walking up to three miles a day, the Kaposi's Sarcoma lesions began to fade, the lymph nodes went down and once more he began to play squash and tennis. Another month and the T4 cell count was a whopping 450. Through Australia's winter and early spring he continued to improve. At this writing the young man feels great and is playing vigorous squash and tennis. He also reports all Kaposi's Sarcoma lesions are gone but one and it is nearly so, swollen lymph nodes are three quarters reduced; the Candida Albicans is almost conquered. He realizes he must stay on his nutrition program to make the recovery complete and to prevent relapses.

There's a tragic postlude to the story: as yet, the young man has not been able to persuade the medical staff at the special hospital trying to cope with AIDS, to treat Candida Albicans in the other AIDS sufferers there! They attribute his progress to good health, a spontaneous remission.

Because we have seen "incurable" diseases recover, we believe virtually all diseases are curable. The same resurgent health that heals tuberculosis or bursitis, asthma or cancer, will heal pneumonia and psoriasis, arthritis and ulcers. The body is no respecter of parts. It will heal them all, given the nutrient repair materials.

ALCOHOLISM: addiction to alcohol.

At birth the stage is set for future alcoholism for millions of Americans with sugar rich formulas instead of mothers' breast milk. The process is continued through childhood and the teen years with white bread, sweet rolls, glazed doughnuts, carbonated drinks, pie, spaghetti, candy, cookies, macaroni, French fries, hot dogs, sugared prepared cereals, and so on. Dr. Roger Williams, in his book *Nutrition Against Disease*, stated categorically that no one who follows good nutritional practices ever becomes an alcoholic. And he has proven that wrong food can create an alcoholic.

Alcoholics frequently report that during a period of low blood sugar they crave alcohol, caffeine, nicotine or sweets. Their recovery has been discouragingly slow, possibly because psychological factors are stressed by physicians while nutritional deficiencies and variables in body chemistry are largely ignored. As do all other cells of the body, brain cells need good nourishment. Diet deficits mean emotional and psychological problems because of brain malfunction from malnutrition. A. Hoffer and H. Osmond, in *Treatment of Schizophrenia Nicotinin Acid or Nicotinomide,* point out that alcoholics and schizophrenics are "kissing kin." They both can have carbohydrate and hormone imbalance from bad diet, wheat-grain allergy and metabolic or functional brain disorder.

A beloved relative of ours suffering from severe alcoholism and agoraphobia did not recover. She was not convinced she should follow an uncomplicated program of no white flour, sugar, coffee, tobacco or alcohol—the real causes of alcoholism—after twice going through a recovery program and staying off alcohol for months. She was only fifty-six when she died.

The rules for our relative were quite simple: Never skip a meal; always eat breakfast. Lunch, the largest and next most important meal, should be the main meal. Dinner should be no more than 500 calories because they will be converted to fat. Snack foods should not contain sugar, chemicals, excess fats or refined carbohydrates. Alcohol, coffee, and smoking were strictly forbidden. These toxic drugs stimulate production of insulin, causing low blood sugar, which in turn, causes such a need for quick energy that the person is driven beyond his or her resistance to consume highly concentrated (processed) carbohydrates.

Meals must include: Protein—lean fish, fowl, fresh raw nuts, sprouted seeds, legumes, cereal grains; carbohydrates—whole grain breads (if grain allergy has been ruled out); fresh fruits; vegetables (not canned); snacks, eaten between meals only if necessary, should be fresh fruits, raw vegetables, nuts, and milk products if tolerated.

Dietary supplements, so very important in the nutrition deficient alcoholic, include all the vitamins and minerals known. A physician should be consulted to determine the specific deficiencies and severity.

An ex-alcoholic friend of ours unable to afford the tests, changed his diet to an all-natural one and took as supplements brewer's yeast, kelp and vitamin C (ten grams a day) and with each gram of vitamin C, 500 milligrams bioflavonoids. He also worked out a good exercise program for *him* at his forty-eight years of age. At this writing he is a young fifty-nine, lean, tanned and strong.

ALLERGIES: Sensitivities to foods and/or substances with resultant reaction.

When foods are digested completely, food allergies rarely exist. Substances the body produces by normal digestion such as amino acids, fruit sugars, glycine, and fatty acids, are never toxic. However, undigested or partly digested foods are toxic. They enter the blood stream when the digestion is subnormal. They act as foreign matter, causing irritation and allergies. For instance, the amino acid histidine from undigested protein may be changed by putrefactive bacteria of the intestines to the toxic substance histamine. Antihistamines are often given to counteract and relieve allergies rather than correcting the cause, which may take a longer time.

Many physicians and biochemists find that most allergies have their start during infancy. Babies are often fed whole cow's milk, meat, cereals, starch, and cooked vegetables from the time they are a few months old. Yet until they are ten to twelve months old their bodies lack the enzymes needed for digesting salted, cooked and complicated nutrients. Cow's milk has much more sodium than mother's milk. This undigested food is in essence poison for the body to throw off and so can cause allergic reactions like skin rashes, colic, etc. Later during childhood and adulthood, countless reactions such as headaches, weakness and fatigue, heart problems, arthritis and hypoglycemia with its multitude of symptoms may result. Other common causes of allergies in our world today are chemical additives in foods, air and water, and the toxic environment from the myriad uses of formaldehyde and polyester clothing, draperies, rugs, upholstery, and from household cleaning solvents.

Alternate therapists have discovered allergies frequently to be the cause of narcolepsy (uncontrollable sleep), insomnia and irritable bowel syndrome. Sometimes they are food allergies, sometimes odors from cleaning and household products, sometimes car odors and sometimes lack of negative ions. All these foods, substances and gaseous odors can be tested by Kinesiology Testing.

An experience with polyester in the early 1970's provided us with a profound insight to its far-reaching harm. We were called to a luxurious new doctor owned hospital some miles away where Elizabeth's sister had just undergone emergency surgery. The glassed in runway to the parking lot was carpeted with polyester, as was the entry room, the elevator to the second floor, the large check in room, the wainscoting, and her sister's room. The odor, a peculiar spicy dust, had seemingly robbed the air of half its oxygen. Elizabeth thought of opening a window for a breath of fresh air but they were hermetically sealed. An air conditioning vent five by twenty inches was the only opening to provide air for two patients, two nurses and several visitors.

Elizabeth greeted her sister who had just regained consciousness and was sipping coffee with milk and nibbling saltine crackers. You can guess our reaction to this fare. All bad—caffeine, milk which is mucous forming and difficult to digest, and white flour crackers containing almost no nutrition except for a few calories. Elizabeth said a few words to her sister, kissed her goodbye, then said to Elton, "Let's go," but no words came out. Elizabeth struggled for balance, for air, for consciousness. Elton and her niece, with a hand under her armpits, helped her out of that maze of carpeted rooms, halls, elevator and runway to fresh air. Elizabeth felt irritable, vicious, evil. If she had had the energy she probably would have committed a crime. As it was, she collapsed on the low wall of the walkway for half an hour, gasping for air and forcing the stale, toxic air out of the lower part of her lungs.

Since that time much human ecology has been learned. Families enclosed in insulated, sealed houses during winter have respiratory infections and become quarrelsome. Nervous and mental problems have been traced to polyester (carpeting for the last several years is made of nylon which is better because it gases off very little), and to formaldehyde in particle board and numerous materials for mobile and motor homes and houses.

Behavior problems can be traced to anything the involved person is exposed to, whether food, air, water or the environment. And his or her reaction can mimic or be the start of almost any degenerative disease.

In contrast to Elizabeth, Elton had few health problems, especially allergies. He didn't seem to have any. But the one he did have was bizarre enough to make up for many.

Bananas were Elton's favorite fruit. He ate them several times a week. Then when we learned how super were frozen, ripe bananas, he ate them every day, just plain or made into fruit ice cream. This was around 1979.

By 1983, Elton was depressed most of the time, antisocial, somewhat paranoid and at times even schizophrenic. He had little energy, no motivation to do anything except to eat and rest because sleep eluded him. He refused to walk the beach, something we like to do every day at our condominium in Mexico.

One day the banana truck drivers went on strike. For five days there were no bananas. Elton never noticed then, but he had enough energy to walk the beach, felt like seeing friends and got back into some research he had started months before. Then the produce truck arrived in front of our condominium. How we enjoyed a lunch of budded sunflower seeds and bananas! Elton ate five or six of them.

Within twenty minutes, he was back into deep depression. No energy. No interest in anything. Although he didn't suspect the problem, Elizabeth did. She hid the bananas so he wouldn't eat one every two or three hours for his low energy and his craving for them. Next morning before breakfast she tested him Kinesiologically. When Elton laid a banana in one hand and extended the other hand and arm for testing, we could feel weakness, not only in the arm but in the whole body. And when she put only a bit of pressure on the wrist to "bounce" the arm for testing the strength, down came Elton's arm. He was shocked. He couldn't believe it. Yet deep down he knew. We felt stupid we hadn't suspected bananas all through the three or four years of worsening health and mental deterioration. Of course, Elton ceased to even touch them.

It took two and one half years of leaving bananas completely alone before he again tested strong while holding one. He ate it with fear and trepidation. Nothing but good happened. However, since learning he does have a tendency to allergic reaction, he doesn't eat them more often than once every four days. And he now goes along with Elizabeth's custom of rotating foods. Elton was hard to convince, but he now knows for certain what havoc allergies can play in a person's life.

ALZHEIMER'S DISEASE: presenile dementia, a degenerative, aging disease beginning most often in persons around fifty years of age.

This tragic disease, on the increase, now affects one in ten people over sixty-five. Aluminum is one of the suspected causes. Vitamin C, the great detoxifier, works effectively to chelate (take) aluminum out of the body. Our nutritionist physician suggests fifteen to twenty grams a day taken in one gram doses every hour along with bioflavonoids including hesperidin and the rest of the bioflavonoid complex (tablet or capsule) that in turn make up the greater vitamin C complex. So far, medical treatments have been basically ineffective.

A few more things have been found by physicians willing to try natural food substances that noticeably alleviate and slow down the inexorable ravages of the problem. They include bee propolis, the B vitamins, acetyl choline, vitamin C and linoleic acid found in unheated plant food oils, in seeds, nuts and avocado. Evening Primrose Oil is held in high esteem by nutrition oriented physicians. It is the richest of all oils thus far researched in the essential fatty acids—gamma lenolenic acid and linoleic acid,—both antiaging foods.

We first became aware of cases of Alzheimer's disease when a distant relative (woman) and a friend of many years (man) were diagnosed as having the "aging" disease, as many then spoke of it. Our relative a few years before, had been diagnosed as having hypoglycemia (low blood sugar). She continued to show many signs of hypoglycemia until her death.

Although our friend seemed in good health, he had vitiligo (white splotches of the skin from depigmentation) when he retired as a telephone engineer. This condition of the skin shows a severe shortage of B vitamins, particularly pantothenic acids and PABA. His twin daughters told us he had for several years complained of constant fatigue. A widower whose beloved wife had died a few years before of heart attack, and a delightful person himself, he became the recipient of well-meaning neighbors who kept him in cookies, cakes, pies and desserts. He lived mostly on these and canned vegetables which lose about half the B vitamins in canning.

Soon he quit driving his car, saying he was too "spooked" to do so. His gait became shuffling, his attention span short, his memory bad. In a few years his daughters, unable to cope with the many facets of his problem, had him cared for in a nursing home where his health deteriorated fast. Until he became incompetent he complained of headache, sleeplessness, fatigue, claustrophobia, aching legs, all classic symptoms of hypoglycemia.

In early September, 1986, we turned on the television to an early morning discussion by an M.D. and a Ph.D. in psychology about Alzheimer's. Each had found a link between the disease and low blood sugar.

Because we were leaving the next day on a 2,800 mile business trip, there was no way we could track down the two men to learn more of what their observations of Alzheimer's had revealed to them. We cannot help but believe that Alzheimer's results not just from aluminum poisoning, however, but also from malnutrition from a conventional diet of canned, prepared and packaged foods, most of which contain chemical additives. In countries of the world where mainly natural foods are eaten the disease is unknown.

Live cell therapy and Rodaquin advocates claim some success in treating the disease as well.

Again, the best thing is to adopt a natural diet and follow a clean, sensible life style to prevent the tragedy of Alzheimer's disease, which seldom occurs in areas where food, water and air are free of processing and pollutants.

ANEMIA: when the blood is deficient in red blood cells, in hemoglobin or in total volume.

The skin of an anemic person is sallow, sometimes grayish and lacking a ruddy glow. So well known is iron deficiency anemia that the many other causes are often overlooked. Treatment with medicinal iron may actually be harmful. Even though iron deficiency is the cause, medicinal iron rarely takes care of the problem, because it isn't readily absorbed. The nutritional approach is found to be the most corrective.

In spite of taking an iron supplement off and on most of her adult life, and at one three-year period by injection, Elizabeth lived with anemia until severe hypoglycemia and an iron, folic acid and B12 deficiency anemia forced her to change her diet. Leaving off processed foods, she ate dark leafy green and colored vegetables such as beet tops and roots, kale, chard, dandelions, comfrey, spinach, broccoli, asparagus, and okra. Other iron-rich vegetables she ate included potatoes, with their peeling, tomatoes, yams and squash. Iron rich fruits she included were dark grapes, apples, plums, apricots, raisins, and bananas. In spite of feeling better, her hemoglobin was little improved after a year. Then Elizabeth read the analysis of spirulina plankton and learned it was about twice as high in vitamin B12 as the next highest food, liver, in this nutrient. She immediately began taking one teaspoonful of the nutrition-packed green algae three times a day. In four weeks her red blood count was high normal. How much improved was her energy! It was almost too good to be true, especially since she was five months into her cancer fight (see Our Personal Stories).

We have observed in our family that no amount of iron, "organic" or inorganic, will be assimilated by the body unless a trace of copper is also in the diet. Absorption was even better when five or six grams of vitamin C (ascorbic acid) were taken each day.

ANOREXIA: loss of appetite.

Anyone who has experienced severe or even mild anorexia knows that much joy of living is gone when food loses its appeal. Whether psychological or physical (preceding, during or following illness), we concentrate on cultivating the appetite by attractive servings of raw fruits and vegetables, nuts and seeds. If cooked foods are decided upon, they should be only those fresh cooked, never canned.

Additives in processed foods tend to add to the anorexia sufferer's aversion to, and disinterest in, eating. But fresh raw fruits and vegetables are cleansing, and when the body is cleansed the appetite tends to return.

ARTHRITIS: inflammation of a joint.

It is quite generally recognized that arthritis, caused by metabolic disturbances, is not a localized disease of certain joints, but a constitutional disease affecting the whole body. A nutritionist-allergist friend of ours says arthritics usually have a too high pH and have too little stomach acid. He finds one to three betaine hydrochloride tablets after meals rectifies this condition. The causes of arthritis can be discovered in overeating, constipation or diarrhea, deficiencies from malnutrition, a sedentary life, physical and emotional stresses, and especially allergies. Adults can test each other for allergies and eliminate those allergen causing foods (see appendix, Kinesiology Testing). These health-ruinous factors result in lowered vitality and resistance to disease, intestinal malabsorption and self-toxicity from poor elimination. In hair analysis, arthritics have been found to have thirty-eight percent more lead than healthy people. Vitamin C helps many to get rid of some lead. And arthritics usually need more manganese, zinc and magnesium. Zinc sulfate topically may improve some types of rheumatoid arthritis.

For many, the don'ts for arthritis are: sugar, white flour, dairy products, citrus fruits, and meat. Faulty digestion of meat often results in uric acid in the tissues. Those are the most allergy causing foods. In Elizabeth's case, the day after she got off white sugar, the constant pain of arthritis in her hands left. That was in 1970 after she had learned she had Addison's disease. For that known killer Elizabeth had just changed to eating mostly raw fruits, seeds, nuts and vegetables, and taking megadoses of vitamin C a day. The wonderful side effect was that over a period of a year or so arthritis in her joints and related soft tissues disappeared completely. Collagen, the "glue" that holds the cells together, has to have ample Vitamin C. Without it there are fibrous tissue accumulations in the joints. Along with toxic wastes and mineral deposits from improperly digested food and from nutrient imbalance, they make up the picture of full-blown arthritis. Orthodox doctors say there is no cure for arthritis. They are right. Their drugs won't cure it. But while they research many are conquering this great crippler through diet (see also JOINT PROBLEMS).

ASTHMA: a condition of labored breathing with wheezing.

Time was when asthma was considered the result mainly of emotional problems. More recently, however, the causes increasingly being discovered are allergies and low blood sugar. It is interesting to note that hypoglycemics are also often asthmatic; diabetics rarely are. When Elton, an asthma sufferer since graduate school days, quit all white sugar, processed foods, social drinking and meat three times a day, asthma quit him. In his case, asthma was mainly a deficiency disease in which he was overfed, overweight and undernourished because of his diet. We have found sugar to be the greatest single cause of asthma.

ATHLETE'S FOOT: a smelly fungus that causes peeling, cracking skin under and between the toes.

Nothing is more annoying than athlete's foot. It thrived on the feet of Elizabeth and those of our number one son until their nutrition was vastly improved, Additionally, they daily bathed the toes in half vinegar and half water, dried them and applied some kind of pure, unprocessed oil. Elizabeth found rendered lamb's fat the best, although her son and others preferred a few drops of crude, raw salad oil from the refrigerator. But the permanent way to deal with toe fungus is to take care of the deficiencies that allowed the fungus to take hold. The B vitamins predominantly are indicated with vitamins A and C close behind. Fungus dislikes them intensely and soon leaves.

AUTISM: a state of mind characterized by daydreaming, hallucinations and disregard of external reality; infantile autism: severe emotional disturbance of childhood characterized by inability to form meaningful interpersonal relationships.

The things that cause autism may cause such abnormalities as hyperactivity, psychiatric depression, childhood schizophrenia and dyslexia.

According to Carl C. Pfeiffer, Ph.D., M.D., in his book *Mental and Elemental Nutrients* (see bibliography), elevated serum (blood) and tissue copper may be as important a factor in autism and other mental problems as is excess lead and mercury.

For years it has been contended that a balanced diet will rid the body of excess toxic minerals. However, there are such differences in quality of soils, fertilizers and foods that it is most difficult to balance a diet in all nutrients, especially minerals. The problem becomes too complicated for a full discussion here, but we would like to relate a few pertinent facts that apply to cases of autism and its correction.

Organically grown foods, lightly cooked or mostly raw are essential. Autistic children appear to need extra taurine, an amino acid. In processed foods, which should be strictly avoided, many vitamins and minerals may be removed or destroyed and extra iron added. This out of balance, excessive mineral may be part of the cause of autism. Excessive copper from copper plumbing, in vitamin-mineral supplements, and copper cooking utensils also seems to contribute to autism. In the case of autism, it is well to consult a nutrition trained physician who can determine mineral imbalances and nutrient deficiencies, and who will plan the necessary all natural foods and supplements for recovery. Happily recovery is not only possible, it is probable.

BAD BREATH: see HALITOSIS.

BALANCE, PROBLEMS OF: the feeling of tilting or leaning of the body; a sensation that you are about to fall.

A largely overlooked micronutrient, manganese, does the lion's share in giving good balance. Shortly after our *UNcook Book* came out, we noticed Elton was falling down now and then, something unusual for him. In a nutrition class a student asked us what manganese was utilized for in the body. Elizabeth remembered the book explained one of the functions is to help the body with proper balance. The very next day Elton started taking it.

In a few weeks, no more falling, even on chuckholed sidewalks and cobblestone streets where we winter in Mexico. Since then, many we've told the manganese story to have been helped. A dear old friend who walked like a tipsy lady for many years, now at 80 has laid aside her cane and walks normally. A young athlete who had been forced to give up basketball is back with his winning team.

We do, however, recommend a consulting a physician if you experience balance problems. There are other causes of imbalance that manganese might not help.

BEDSORES: abscesses on the skin resulting from severe malnutrition and prolonged confinement in bed

There is no excuse for allowing bedsores to develop. Patients suffering this problem of neglect are woefully deficient in many nutrients, especially zinc, vitamins A, E, B2 and C. Vitamins A and E are useful to heal the sores. Bedsore patients invariably have a high pH. Immediate effort should be made to get the pH lowered to 5.5 to keep the bacteria of the sores from multiplying. This may be done quite rapidly by giving two to three betain hydrochloride tablets after meals, prunes, cranberry juice, and two to three teaspoons of apple cider vinegar in water with a little honey added. Raw honey and vitamin C water (put two grams C powder in six ounces of water) should be applied to the sores. The diet should immediately be made optimal, mostly uncooked or slightly cooked.

BED-WETTING (enuresis): urinating in bed, especially involuntarily and habitually.

Bed-wetting is a problem all too common in early childhood, sometimes in early adulthood and commonly occurring in the aging. Some causes have been stated as psychological problems, overstrenuous toilet training, nutritional deficiencies and allergy. Of the several cases of bed-wetting in children and adults within our family and friends, all have been completely relieved in a matter of days when the missing nutrients of magnesium, vitamin B2 and pantothenic acid were given, the calcium intake lowered, and allergy causing food was removed from the diet. The bed-wetter has a smaller bladder capacity because the detrusor muscle is in spasm, a manifestation of an allergy (see appendix, Kinesiology Testing).

Years ago Elizabeth had bladder control trouble. Until TV commercials alerted her to the universality of the problem, she had forgotten that dilemma. For her own magnesium deficiency, an allergist friend advised Elizabeth to take unflavored milk of magnesia. (She has since changed to magnesium citrate which is more readily assimilated.) However, it is easy to regulate the dose of milk of magnesia precisely. For children she suggests one half teaspoon in water or juice two or three times a day preferably between meals; for adults, one teaspoon. Elizabeth ate foods rich in pantothenic acid and vitamin B2 such as sprouts of all kinds, soaked nuts, spirulina plankton, brewer's yeast and bee pollen. She also took cinnamon bark tea. It is really better to chew a piece of bark since cinnamon bark is not only a fair source of minerals and B vitamins, but has a factor that is especially good for urine control. People not completely helped by magnesium may need to take one to three potassium chloride tablets a day in addition.

BEE STING: Last summer Elton came running in from gardening with seven red bee sting welts suddenly raised to the size of quarters. He took eight grams of ascorbic acid. In a few minutes the welts were receding and the pain was gone. In a few hours nothing was visible except the tiny wounds where the stingers pierced the skin. After an application or two of vitamin E, they were gone the next morning.

Everyone we know of who has taken ascorbic acid has had the same results: three grams in the case of children; six or eight grams for adults. Our handyman, so allergic to bee sting he'd been hospitalized with severe toxicity several times, was stung by our belligerent bees last year. But after eight grams of vitamin C powder and ten minutes of incredulously observing his welts disappear, he went back to work muttering something about a confounded miracle.

BEHAVIOR PROBLEMS: Unnatural or abnormal behavior.

In scientific journals and the news media, there's an ever-increasing number of reports linking unnatural or abnormal behavior in children, teenagers, adults, mental patients and prisoners to nutritional deficiencies, allergies to foods, additives in foods, chemicals in water and air, petrochemicals in clothing, household furnishings, building materials, cleaning products, and so on. By count, some 10,000 chemicals are in use in the world today. Those chemicals tend to rob our bodies of vitamins and minerals, especially vitamin C, magnesium and calcium.

When people are free from allergy-causing foods, polluted air and water, and away from synthetics, they are relaxed, calm and more even tempered. On the contrary, chemically loaded foods, working or sleeping in a particle board room, a few minutes at a filling station to get gas and they may feel cross and irritable. For some, a visit to the dry cleaners may cause near panic.

Before Elizabeth overcame cancer she got a headache from latex paint. An interior of polyester carpeting and drapes robbed the enclosure of much oxygen, burnt her sinuses, made her feel evil, and drained her of energy. Were it not for ensuing confusion, loss of speech and severe weakness, she feared she could have committed violence.

Our three-year-old grandson demonstrated what sugar and/or additives in foods can do to a child's behavior. At a restaurant he was given the red maraschino cherries from his parents' cocktails, his own "cocktail" of ginger ale, and white flour crackers to munch on. When dinner was served, he refused anything but a bit of milk and a bite of bleached flour roll. By the time dinner was over he was quarrelsome. When we went for a drive he was incorrigible. His parents were completely nonplused at his unusual behavior until a few days later when they read a report on the "probable" cause of hyperactive children: sugar and food additives. One typically well behaved little boy from then on got very little sugar and few additives.

Not only do chemicals, either singly or in numbers, directly and indirectly, cause a multitude of illnesses, they play havoc with our nervous system and brain. One of the most common reactions of the body to their ingestion, breathing, or body contact is a shortened supply of glycogen (body starch) that the liver stores for emergency. If it is in short supply, the brain and nervous system cannot efficiently do their job of maintaining body calm, mind balance and emotional stability. The shorter the supply of glycogen, or blood sugar as it is called when in the veins and being distributed all over the body, the more "berserk" the brain and nervous system become.

Allergens from any source, as foods, drugs, odors, materials, etc., can also cause low blood sugar. When the chemicals are removed and the body allowed to recuperate, performance is normal. The individual is not "uptight." Tension, overactivity, restlessness, irritability and ill temper fade away. Vitamin C, a powerful detoxifier, calcium and magnesium all have a calming effect on the hyperactive child or adult.

While Elizabeth was testing foods after the diagnostic fast in the hospital, workmen were applying hot asphalt on the parking lot outside her window. The fumes gave her such a headache she could not eat. She felt extremely cross, argumentative and hateful. By midmorning she was drained of energy. We learned that her blood sugar had plummeted to fifty. The odors of a dry cleaning establishment and a filling station used to do the same thing. Candles heavily scented with petroperfumes gave her a disagreeable "high" of spite filled energy, soon followed by fatigue.

All petrochemicals are toxic. Harmless looking mineral oil and vaseline block the body's use of oil soluble vitamins (A, B, D, K) and vitamin C. Stated more bluntly, they destroy those essential vitamins. Yet a body rub that is universally used by hospitals, on babies and for complexions is mainly mineral oil scented with petro-perfume. On a test exposure to polyester (clothing, drapes, upholstery, carpeting) in the fasting clinic, Elizabeth had a real psychedelic trip, pleasant and fascinating at the time, but which drained her energy for hours, a time when she passed through all sorts of negative emotions as irritability, depression, anger, vindication. As her body threw off all the toxins and she was back to normal, she again felt good-humored, joyous and optimistic.

We cannot help but feel there should be more reports of studies made on what poisons in food, air and water do to the nervous system and behavior. What if a young person, say a teenager, got a reaction similar to Elizabeth's from polyester? If he or she felt as evil as Elizabeth did and had energy, what might have happened? Vandalism from frustration? Murder from deep-seated resentment?

When the food in penal institutions has been greatly improved, so has the behavior and attitude of the inmates. Why are our conventional professionals so reluctant to consider and try this simple, inexpensive method of improving behavior? It could help empty our correctional and mental institutions. It makes such sense. It is so natural.

BLEMISHES: see FACIAL SIGNS OF HEALTH PROBLEMS and ACNE

BLOOD POISONING: see GANGRENE

BONE PROBLEMS: osteoporosis or porous, shrunken bones; weak undeveloped bones in children.

Osteoporous, usually in people over fifty, is generally caused by nutritional deficiencies, lack of exercise, medications such as cortisone, improper utilization and absorption of nutrients, post menopausal hormonal imbalances, and eating too much meat.

In wild animals, bones increase in density and strength with age. Scrimshaw artists and craftspeople prefer bones from old wild animals. Their bones are dense. In today's humans the opposite is true. Prolonged deficiencies in calcium and vitamin D—lack of sunshine—along with insufficient magnesium, phosphorous, hydrochloric acid and vitamin C, bring on this condition. Although bones within a few hours will start to improve once the person is on an adequate diet, it may take a few years to reach normal density.

After years of illness, immobility and a conventional diet which at best was inadequate to maintain good health, the doctor X-rayed her chest when Elizabeth recovered from a back injury. The bones of her rib cage were like Swiss cheese, full of holes that indicated great calcium loss. About that time our nutrition-practicing physician helped us with an optimal diet for the colon cancer Elizabeth was trying to conquer. It included brewer's yeast, spirulina plankton, megadoses of vitamin C, sesame seeds which are extremely high in calcium, fish liver oil, vitamin D (1,000 units a day), outdoor walks, sunbaths when possible, and a quart of shave grass (horsetail) tea a day. In this case the all-natural diet for cancer was right for osteoporous. He said the silicon rich tea, the highest known plant in silica, had helped his osteoporosis patients to recover quicker by far than any nutrition regimen without it. Certainly it worked for Elizabeth. An X-ray of her jaw after minor surgery three years later showed very dense bone, and her backache had ceased. We must add that during most of these years Elizabeth did exercises, even though limited much of the time because of low energy.

Some doctors believe there is no cure of osteoporosis. Yet bones are made up of living cells which are known to do an excellent job of repair and maintenance if sufficient calcium, magnesium, phosphorous, potassium, vitamin D, and vitamin C and, in lesser amounts, all other vitamins and minerals in natural foods are provided. Dark green leafy vegetables, full of minerals, must not be neglected. If they are cooked, the cooking liquid which contains a lot of the minerals, should be eaten. Older patients on a high protein diet develop osteoporosis while older vegetarians do not. To keep your good bones or to restore the missing nutrients, plan your nutrition to meet all body needs, do daily vigorous exercise, get some sun each week, then praise and thank God for the health and healing He has for you.

BRONCHITIS: an inflammation of the air passages to the lungs.

Such factors as respiratory diseases (emphysema, asthma), air pollution, fatigue, chilling, cigarette smoking, malnutrition, chronic staphylococcus infections, and low resistance can all lead to susceptibility to bronchitis. Symptoms often start with sore throat, fever, muscle and back pain, fatigue and/or a dry cough that develops into one that brings up mucus as the inflammation increases.

Many years ago Elizabeth acquired staphylococcus infection of the sinus while hospitalized. With a low immune system from having been given an antibiotic that partially destroyed the bone marrow years before, plus conventional diet and resulting malnutrition, she was unable to conquer it. Not until several years after getting over many diseases including colon cancer did she improve her health enough to finally rid her body of the staph infection of the sinus that had long before spread to a spot in the upper bronchial tubes.

Here is the program that finally allowed Elizabeth to surmount the problem that made her susceptible to lung and bronchial pneumonia, colds and flu: an all-raw diet for maximum nutrition, fiber for continuous cleansing and for plenty of oxygen to all cells; elimination of all food allergens and all possible air, water and fabric pollutants by Kinesiological

Testing (see appendix, Kinesiology Testing). She began daily walks in clean air, summer and winter, plus vigorous exercise such as push-ups, slow leg-lifts while lying on the floor and five minutes of deep breathing exercises. Wearing layers of clothing including a triple fold of cotton flannel over the upper chest (thymus) against chilling enabled her to be able to add or take off enough to maintain the same body temperature. She also did morning and evening sinus irrigation for triggering a deep cough to bring up the small, stiff, ropy staph infection (pus) that imbeds in bronchial pockets.

Here are directions for sinus irrigation, which is a painless treatment: In eight ounces of sterilized water, dissolve one half teaspoon sodium ascorbate powder and one pinch of sea salt. With the index finger on left hand, hold left nostril tightly closed. Hold glass of water tightly up to nose and "drink" it in the right nostril to a slow count of seven. Tilt back the head. You may cough spontaneously before you get a chance to allow the soothing liquid to go farther back in the throat. Try again and again. You'll learn how to control the coughing with practice. After two or three times "drinking" the liquid with each nostril (a time or two with one side, then with the other), blow your nose to clear out the mucous. Then proceed again until all the water in the glass is gone (a total of ten or twelve "drinks"). Elizabeth rarely got out the small pus globs on the first few coughs. As the induced coughing gets deeper with each irrigation, more and sometimes all, accumulated infection is coughed up. If not, you'll soon know it from having to persistently clear your throat. Before rehearsals and performances, we have demonstrated this technique to speakers and singers who have the problem of throat clearing from sinus and/or chronic bronchial infections, a twice-a-day chore that, they report, has helped them immeasurably. And after much urging, we demonstrated the sinus irrigation technique to a lecture audience of doctors in Amsterdam who are teaching their patients to assume the responsibility for their own health and ways to help themselves.

Another sinus irrigation solution that is equally effective and some doctors say even more soothing is a ten percent solution of table sugar. To make, dissolve all sugar possible into distilled or boiled water. Dissolve one part of this solution in nine parts of boiled or distilled water. When we use this solution, we make up a gallon at a time for convenience.

Note: During the first two or three times of douching the nostril, you may spontaneously cough before you can pull water well into the sinus, for postnasal mucous may be loosened and cause the expelling cough. For a few minutes after the irrigation, you may have a watery nose and some throat clearing. However, soon your nostrils, sinuses and throat will feel marvelously free and clean.

BRUISES, SPONTANEOUS (SB): a descriptive phrase denoting a bruise occurring without a known cause.

Spontaneous bruising is another "small" affliction, a symptom of deficiency so common today mostly among those over forty, but increasingly occurring in young adults and even children.

Spontaneous bruises appear most often on arms and legs. Elizabeth had this illusive, mysterious problem for years before she learned it was B2, C and E vitamin deficiencies. Bioflavonoids also play a part, especially for oxygen to the injured cells and for healing. There are usually other deficiencies too. If SB people do not eat enough fresh, uncooked foods to meet their needs for vitamins, it may mean they are also not getting enough of the other vitamins, minerals and enzymes to maintain good health. It clearly appears that nutrition is the major answer to ending spontaneous bruising.

BUNION: swelling and extreme tenderness of the joint of the big toe.

Although bunions may be caused by an inherited weakness of the foot bone, muscles or ligaments, it usually results from wearing shoes too short, tapered or small.

The best way to treat bunions is to prevent them by wearing rounded toe shoes large enough to give room for the toes without crowding. In severe cases of bunions, surgery may be necessary. However, most bunions can be helped by properly fitted, low heel shoes.

The pain, the soreness, the swelling of bunions can be relieved by placing the feet in a foot bath of one gallon of lukewarm (not hot) water in which five or six teaspoons of vitamin C powder have been dissolved. Leave the feet in the water until it cools to room temperature. This will take forty-five to sixty minutes. Do this foot bath therapy morning and night for two or three days or until the pain and tenderness in the big toe joints are gone. It is necessary during and after the treatment to wear well fitting, low heel, comfortable shoes.

BURNS: thermal, sunburn and X-ray.

Burns respond to a number of different treatments. Immediately immerse the burn in very cold water or run cold water over the area until the "heat" and pain leaves. Then treat by applying vitamin E, aloe vera gel, fresh juice from aloe vera leaves or liquid honey to completely cover the burned area. Take vitamin C orally. Also vitamin C dissolved in water and sprayed on the skin is a treatment found to be most effective for severe burns.

We have employed all these treatments depending on what is readily available or suitable in coping with emergencies happening to ourselves and others. In winter, friends who visit us in our beach condominium, in spite of our many warnings, invariably get a severe sunburn. We've given a starch bath (two cups cornstarch to a tub full of water) or a vinegar bath (two cups apple cider vinegar in a tub full of water). Both are very soothing. After the bath we gently rub the skin with vitamins E and A mixed with olive oil or other vegetable oil. In the refrigerator we keep a mixture of a tablespoon each of cold pressed avocado oil, almond oil, olive oil, 1,000 IU of vitamin E and 50,000 IU of vitamin A with a drop of perfume, not only for emergency sunburn, but for the complexion.

In case of burn wound infection, nothing works more magically than packing the affected area with white sugar three or four times a day after washing out the wound with hydrogen peroxide. Dressings are painless and easy to dress. They do not stick to the wound. Doctors say sugar tends to soak up moisture, thus causing bacteria to "die of thirst." Richard A. Knutson, M.D. of Delta Medical Center, Greenville, Mississippi, mixes one quart iodine ointment from the drug store and four parts sugar. He has used this ointment on cut, scrape, and burn wounds of some 2,245 patients with great results. Wounds heal almost entirely without scars.

BURSITIS: Inflammation of the burse, a sac-like cavity of the shoulder.

For two years this severe inflammation nearly incapacitated Elizabeth's left arm. Cortisone and other medications did nothing to relieve it. But when she quit sugar and all processed

foods to get over Addison's disease, the bursitis disappeared as
steadily as a puddle of water in warm sunshine.

Elizabeth has since learned that chloride rich foods (which
she had just begun to eat and continues to eat regularly) such as
avocado, tomatoes, kelp, endive, celery, oats, and watercress
eaten raw, are beneficial. Oats should be soaked overnight, then
warmed over a pan of hot, not boiling, water. They may be
served with a bit of butter and honey. We praise the Lord for
this delicious, inexpensive, natural food full of the best kind of
soothing fiber.

CANCER: a tumorous, malignant growth or area of radical,
malignant cell proliferation.

The sinister assassin, cancer, now kills one person in four.
Yet it is not necessary, we firmly believe, for people to die from
this dread disease.

There is much evidence to substantiate that cancer is a
deficiency disease. It is shocking to realize that the great cancer
research centers ignore this well-founded observation. They
study the end result of this problem, the cancer, and seek to
eliminate or kill it. Yet cancer is a *symptom* of greatly
deteriorated health of the whole body through malnutrition,
abuse, pollution, etc. Many noted therapists, scientists and
physicians as Dr. Linus Pauling, Dr. Richard Cathcart, and Dr.
Jeffery Bland find that vitamin C is one of the key nutrients in
prevention and recovery from cancer. Vitamin D is another.

We personally know of many who were healed after they
went on an all-raw diet. They include a woman with throat
cancer, and another with colon and rectal cancers. A college
roommate of years ago, had bone cancer completely arrested by
a mostly raw diet and Laetrile; the uncle of a Mexican professor
friend conquered prostate cancer with "la comida vivienda,"
living foods, as he says. And we know of a number of other
victors here, in Australia, in Mexico and in Europe who
eliminated cancer from their bodies by a completely raw diet.
Dr. Christine Nolfi of Denmark, after eliminating her own
breast cancer with an all-raw diet, set up a clinic and health spa
and cured many people of cancer with organically grown, raw
foods. She became world famous for her dedicated work.

Twice, years before Elizabeth changed her health-destroying
eating and living habits, she had radical cells in the cervix. After
changing to a raw diet, she had no more such problems.

Biochemical researchers have discovered that radical and cancerous cells appear in a body that hasn't sufficient enzymes for adequate food absorption, especially animal protein. Without adequate absorption the body is left deficient in many ways and vulnerable to any or all degenerative diseases. Such was her case.

Why an all-raw diet? We're glad you asked. Here are some reasons: none of the nutrition is destroyed, lost or altered. Vitamins, minerals, enzymes, proteins, fats, carbohydrates—all intact—can serve their purpose to their maximum, as God intended. From thirty to eighty-five percent of the nutrients are destroyed in cooking, an overall average of fifty percent. The body gets full benefit of the nourishment in living foods, the highest quality of building and repair supplies for growth, for health maintenance and repair of disease damage. A person with the will to get over cancer cannot afford to put a single bite into his or her mouth that is not health giving.

There is no neutral ground for food. They either give us energy/health or they take away energy/health. Cells have to have oxygen. Cooking, firing, heating destroy the oxygen. Remember this recognized fact: cancer cells cannot proliferate where cells get enough oxygen. In other words, cancer works only in unhealthy, oxygen-starved, undernourished places in the body. Man is the only animal that fires his food and man is the most disease-wracked of all creatures. The correlation between meat eating and the incidence of cancer has been established. Overeating of animal protein, especially muscle meat, overworks the pancreas, causing insufficiency of pancreatic enzymes which are necessary for protein metabolism. This unmetabolized protein putrefies in the gut and is reabsorbed, making poisoned blood that starts and contributes to disease.

Cancer patients are found to be deficient in the trace mineral selenium (abundant in yeast), and vitamin C. Many getting over cancer take twenty to thirty grams a day around the clock, then ten grams a day after recovery or for cancer prevention. Fish oil vitamin A is also very valuable, some physicians prescribe 50,000 to 75,000, even 100,000 IU a day for cancer recovery; 10,000 to 25,000 IU a day for maintenance.

Too much iron in the system, either from an iron-high diet (rare) or iron supplements can contribute to the growth of cancer. Cancer cells and bacteria *have* to have iron to proliferate. One of the very real hidden dangers of processed foods is the ferrous sulfate and several iron compounds that are used as supplements, substances that are rarely metabolized properly by the body and cause harm by destroying vitamin E (known since 1928), carotene and vitamins A and C. They greatly increase the need for several nutrients as pantothenic acid and oxygen. Iron salts given during pregnancy have been found to cause miscarriages, deformities in the baby, mental retardation or defect, and susceptibility to anemia and jaundice. All these dangers were pointed out in medical journals in the 1950's and 1960's.

Despite this knowledge and much more since then, the food industry still uses iron supplements (medicinal iron) in refined products. At a cost of millions for advertising, pharmaceuticals and multivitamin manufacturers keep the specter of "iron-poor blood," especially for women, before the public and many doctors still prescribe iron.

Small wonder Elizabeth had cancer and chronic infection with all the ferrous sulfate, the iron shots, the iron compounds she took over a twenty-five year period following the instructions of doctors. Iron *feeds* cancer and the bacteria of infection. After recovering from cancer on an all-raw diet, Elizabeth was still anemic. However, she soon learned about spirulina plankton. After taking one teaspoon three times a day for three and one-half weeks, her hemoglobin was high normal. On an all-raw diet with plenty of sprouted seeds, grains and legumes, she maintains very healthy blood.

We agree with many who now believe that cancer treatment must begin with elimination of the causes—environmental sources of such carcinogens as smoking, radiation, and chemicals in food, water and air, along with correcting food deficiencies. Elizabeth did all this.

In a little over two years Elizabeth overcame colon cancer and skin cancers. Through the course of twenty-two months, stumbling, bumbling, trial and error, Elizabeth did it all because God did not leave her. Through prayer, persistance and patience, He accomplished in her what others had dismissed as her folly. When God leads and we follow, miracles occur.

CANDIDA ALBICANS INFECTION: a yeastlike overgrowth chiefly in the gastrointestinal tract and vagina.

Ordinarily Candida albicans obtains its nourishment from dead organic matter, performing a scavenger service for the body. Normally it is balanced by beneficial flora. But when antibiotics are used too much this good flora is killed, upsetting the balance and allowing the Candida to increase. This overgrowth gives rise to colitis, esophagitis and vaginitis.

Candida albicans overgrowth moves in when our immune system is low, when our body is debilitated by a deficiency of nutrients, when the system is weakened for whatever reason, after a period of taking antibiotics, corticosteroids, birth control pills, or large amounts of sugar which paralyzes the phagocytic capacity of our white blood cells. Likewise, lack of sleep, lack of meticulous hygiene, chronic constipation or diarrhea, the irritative chemicals we breathe, anxiety, chronic food-chemical allergies or too much physical stress, can bring it on. Underlying these possible causes are unmet needs for specific nutrients which must be tested, then satisfied, before improvement is made in conquering Candida.

There are drugs for treatment but they do not cure metabolic and nutrient deficiencies, the initial cause of the illness. If nutritional needs are not met, the overgrowth continues and disease after disease follows, becoming worse with time.

The person who suffers Candida albicans needs to find a physician practicing nutrition to overcome it. Several years ago when Elizabeth's mouth, esophagus and intestinal tract suddenly broke out in ulcerated fungus (Candida) after three weeks of antibiotics for near fatal pneumonia, the lung specialist said, "That apple cider vinegar you've been taking: now it will be useful." He had been called in when her doctor, an allergist-pediatrician, said, "This is too much pneumonia for a pediatrician." The lung man had insisted she take a mixture of antibiotics in spite of her being allergic to several of them. He had agreed to allow her doctor to give her eighty grams daily of vitamin C intravenously and include the antibiotics in the C solution. Because nobody really thought she'd live, they did not contest her taking a daily dose of seventy grams of vitamin C and many teaspoons a day of vinegar the allergist-pediatrician provided. He had wanted to give Elizabeth 150 grams of vitamin C a la Philpott, proven for healing pneumonia in two or three days, but the hospital doctors would not permit it.

Elizabeth's body pH was so high on the alkaline side it was frightening. But soon after the intensive care stage, blood transfusion and lung taps, she began to show improvement. After three weeks of the antibiotics, when Candida (ulcerated fungus) broke out, nystatin was given to her. It helped, perhaps, but soon the hospital and drug store's supply ran out. Elizabeth continued with megadoses of vitamin C as her allergist/physician recommended. After her six weeks stay in the hospital, at her allergist's suggestion, she took lactobacillus acidophilus, olive oil (one tablespoon a day for oleic acid and/or biotin), the yolk of a two-minute soft-boiled egg and three tablespoons primary yeast daily.

She improved steadily, recovering her strength, overcoming the hideous cough, and gaining weight weeks ahead of the lung specialist's prediction. When he later learned of her remarkable recovery, he said, "Some things that happen I do not understand." Our pediatrician-allergist physician and loving friend understands. So do we.

CANKER SORES: abscesses in the mouth.

When the body's resistance is lowered, there's usually an extra need for all nutrients. One especially needed for canker sores we find is the B3 vitamin, niacin. It's high in brewer's yeast. One of the times we may develop a canker sore is during travel when stress may be great and foods wrong. However, extra niacin (or niacinamide), vitamin A, the B vitamins, especially B6 which we get in yeast and/or spirulina plankton, and vitamin C (ascorbic acid), heal them for us in a day or two. Vitamin C water (one gram vitamin C dissolved in one half cup water and held in the mouth a few minutes) will relieve canker sores and start their healing. Remember that for this mouth wash, vitamin C as *sodium ascorbate* is better for repeated treatments. It does not affect the teeth as does ascorbic acid which tends to dissolve the enamel.

CATARACTS: thickening of the lens of the eye.

According to research done by eight ophthalmologists with over a thousand patients in England several years ago, and reported in *Science Magazine,* the single greatest cause of cataracts was the body's inability to cope with food sugars. At the top of the list was milk sugar (lactose) with refined white sugar next. Since that time many eye specialists have noted that the diet of the majority of cataract patients includes a substantial amount of dairy products and refined white sugar. Cataracts can also develop when the diet is inadequate and prolonged stress is endured.

When Elizabeth was at the bottom of the health scale, in 1965, the ophthalmologist found early stage cataracts in her eyes. Being an orthodox physician, he had no words of wisdom on what to do to slow or stop their development. In reading what several nutritionists of that day had to say about cataracts, however, Elizabeth decided to put more emphasis on the fairly natural diet we had worked out at that time. We read the report of the research the ophthalmologists had done in England. As time went on and we learned more, Elizabeth gave up all processed foods, took extra potassium chloride for a discovered serum deficiency of it, and lived on mostly raw foods.

When Elizabeth learned a few years later that she had cancer of the ascending colon (one of the slow growing kinds of tumor), and went on a completely raw diet to conquer it, her eyes further improved. In the nine years since the cancer diagnosis and the all-living foods diet, our eye specialist continues to report "a very slight beginning" of cataract. On the correct diet for *her,* many illnesses and problems have disappeared. This one may too.

CHELATION: another modality for clearing arteries, as for heart trouble.

Although not banned, intravenous chelation is "under the gun." Chelation, many conventional physicians realize, has made heart bypass surgery obsolete, yet this drastic operation brings in such revenue that many doctors and hospitals would face economic disaster if it were discontinued.

The dictionary explains: "chelate: of, relating to or having a cyclic structure usually containing five or six atoms in a ring in which a central metalic ion is held in a coordination complex." The verb chelate is from the Greek word that means *to grab onto.* The chelating substance, usually EDTA, given intravenously in a two to three hour drip, grabs onto toxic metals and carries them, via the blood stream, through the body's elimination system and out. At the same time it takes out obstructing deposits, thus clearing the blood vessels for good circulation and normal heart function. Another method of chelation, effective for many, is carefully planned nutrition and supplementation after the individual patient's needs have been determined by tests.

Although chelation rids the body of toxic metals, it also takes out other metals needed for metabolism. To rectify this situation, nutrients necessary for health are added to the i.v. solution to maintain mineral stability.

The treatment for obstructed arteries is one to three a week continuing several weeks or even months. From the first few treatments the patient begins to feel better and continues to improve until the physician finds the arteries clean. At this time, the patient is feeling good, his weight has usually come down to normal for him, his diet is vastly improved and highly nutritious, he's capable of vigorous activity and he is inexpressibly joyous. He is so grateful he tells all who listen.

CHLORINE and FLUORIDE: for purposes of this book, two chemicals put in public water supplies, the former to kill bacteria, the latter to prevent tooth decay.

A word of warning: both chlorine and fluoride destroy vitamins when taken into the body. They are known to be carcinogenic and toxic (poisonous). The incidence of cancer rises sharply after chlorine is added, and really climbs when both it and fluoride are added to a city's water supply. By setting aside a widemouth jar or pitcher of water for a few hours, most of the chlorine will evaporate. Not so with fluoride. It is there to stay.

Putting fluoride in toothpaste is a tragic mistake. The small amount of this poison, used day in, day out, twice a day, is readily absorbed through the tissues of the mouth. Remember, it is toxic. *It is cumulative.* That means it *stays* in the body. Over a period of time, it subtly begins to cause a problem. The muscles of most of us test weak when we barely touch a bit of toothpaste. Our own reaction to using toothpaste with fluoride is less energy and, for Elizabeth, a redness on the eyelids. Think what it does to small children who are allowed to use a great glob of it, then take a lot of time to brush their teeth while parents compliment them for doing a good job. Fluoride toothpaste, besides fluoride, may have artificial color and artificial sweetener, both toxins.

Swimming pools are many times so chlorinated that some people can't go in them, especially indoor ones. Not only does the skin absorb chlorine, the lungs take it into the body. Janitors and maintenance people of such facilities are often quite susceptible to colds and flu, low energy and headaches. Chlorine has been linked to anemia, high blood pressure, cholesterol, atherosclerosis and its end results, heart attack and stroke.

Hydrogen peroxide is an excellent substitute for keeping pools free from bacteria and contagion. It costs only a little. There is no health ravage from it. Investigate and try it.

The side effects of fluoride are several and scary. It is not volatile as is chlorine. It not only destroys vitamin C, it can cause liver and kidney damage. All this is the price many thousands of people in the United States pay for the privilege (?) of allowing their children and themselves to eat candy and other sweets, and, they think, suffer less tooth decay.

Pure water is almost nonexistent in America today. Even though with chlorinated water there is relatively little danger of contracting cholera or typhoid, there is real danger of swallowing lead, mercury, chloroform, carbon tetrachloride, arsenic, pesticides, rust, dead bacteria, pipe debris, and more.

Pure food and water God provided for in the natural state give energy and maintain health. Chemically contaminated food and water *destroy* energy and health.

CHOLESTEROL PROBLEMS: cholesterol, a crystaline fatty alcohol, an essential nutrient.

When we see or hear the word, we think of the cholesterol in animal fats that we may eat, or the cholesterol in eggs or shellfish.

Cholesterol is necessary to the life of every cell. Whether or not we ingest cholesterol-containing foods, our body tissues synthesize it from carbohydrates. If those carbohydrates are highly refined (sugar and white flour), the cholesterol particles will be too large to readily go in and out of the cell walls. When there is sticky plaque on the artery walls from the wrong kinds of fats, those large cholesterol deposits stick to the fatty plaque. Thus begins atherosclerosis.

What causes the sticky plaque? Recent findings point to hydrogenated oils and fats (grocery cooking oils and margarine with a shelf life of almost *forever* that have no vitamin E left in them).

The ideal diet to prevent cholesterol build up is one of unrefined foods containing all essential nutrients. When vitamins A and E and the essential oils found in such cold pressed ones as safflower, soy, peanut and sesame, and all seeds and nuts, are contained in the food supply, there is no sticky plaque in the arteries and cholesterol deposits and gallstones are not a problem. While orthodox medicine largely ignores all this, many people are bringing down cholesterol levels to normal, ridding their arteries of sticky plaque and dissolving gallstones which are mainly cholesterol. Cold pressed olive oil is effective in helping to lower cholesterol deposits.

Elton had high blood pressure and high cholesterol from graduate school days until he went on a completely unrefined diet with no sugar, white flour, or processed oils and fats. (Lecithin, from soy, helps to bring down cholesterol levels and blood pressure.) He eats three soft boiled eggs twice a week and occasionally shrimp. His blood pressure is 130/72 and his cholesterol is 140. Elizabeth's blood pressure is 118/70 and her cholesterol 130.

Cholesterol is not a problem for the all-natural food eater.

CLAUSTROPHOBIA: inordinate fear of close enclosures.

Hypoglycemics are often sufferers of phobias. Elizabeth endured claustrophobia, the fear and confusion of things too close around. Another member of our family suffered agoraphobia, the fear of open spaces. Once the hypoglycemia was corrected by elimination of allergies and by natural diet, the phobias were gone. Muscle testing can help you find your allergies. Eliminate those offending foods, improve your nutrition and your phobia may quickly disappear.

COLD EXTREMITIES: chronically cold hands and feet.

Poor circulation, small veins and arteries, low blood volume, heart problems, nutritional deficiencies, hypothroidism, nervous disorder and lack of exercise are all conducive to cold hands and feet.

Vigorous exercise, reflexology and the raw foods Elizabeth chose for getting over all sort of illnesses noticeably helped in every way except, she has to confess, with cold hands and feet. It is generally accepted by orthomolecular physicians that niacin, RN (ribo-nucleic acid), vitamins B2, E and C alleviate the problem that she still has somewhat. She has not taken extra nucleic acid (bought at health food stores). It might be worth a try.

COLDS: a respiratory viral infection characterized by sneezing, sore throat, running nose, and coughing.

Many have heard of or read *Vitamin C and the Common Cold,* by Dr. Linus Pauling. We can only say that one should try vitamin C in the amount and way he suggests when feeling the onset of a cold or flu. We suggest taking a maintenance dose sufficient to prevent the onset (three to six grams a day at intervals).

We find the addition of vitamin A and a little apple cider vinegar highly beneficial. (Two teaspoons in a glass of water after meals.) When we take all three supplements regularly—vitamin A, vitamin C, and apple cider vinegar—we're rarely threatened by a cold or flu.

Prunes, cranberries and blueberries are also great to help ward off or get over a cold. Cherries, peaches, apples, apricots and grapes are good too. Why these fruits, especially cranberries, blueberries and apple cider vinegar? They help the body to get from the alkaline to the acid side. Bacteria and viruses cannot multiply in an acid environment. The acid-alkaline balance in the body is called pH, and is indicated by running a little urine over a piece of nitrozene paper the first thing on arising. (see appendix, "pH") The number 7.0 on the pH scale is neutral. Slightly acid is ideal—6.5 to 5.0. When we get up in the morning, feeling great, and check our pH, we invariably find it to be 5.0 or 5.5, which is slightly acid. If we are ill, our pH is 7.0 or higher. Remember that all people ill with infection, bacterial or virus, suffer a high pH. Well people have a lower pH which means their bodies are slightly acid. It is nature's way of protecting us from infection. The mantle (outer covering) of the skin is slightly acid. If it weren't, our bodies would be vulnerable to the millions of bacteria and viruses that touch us constantly.

At the first sign of a sore throat, take a clean washcloth, napkin or handkerchief, stick out your tongue, grasp it tightly and pull up, down, sideways and at angles as far as possible, once each way. This stimulates the sluggish lymph glands, starts the flow of lymph, and stimulates blood circulation. In a few minutes the soreness of the throat will have lessened or disappeared. But don't stop there. Your body's resistance has been lowered—that is, fatigued, chilled, overfed, suffered emotional upset or whatever—and you must do more.

At such a time your body is under stress. In this early stage the adrenal glands may not be able to produce the hormone *aldosterone* that holds salt in the tissues. This salt is spilled through the urine. A drop on the end of the tongue can tell you if you are spilling salt. When this happens to us, we immediately take our cold prevention cocktail: three teaspoons apple cider vinegar, one eighth to one fourth teaspoon sea salt, one fourth teaspoon honey, three grams ascorbic acid powder, stirred into a ten-ounce glass of water and sipped with a straw to keep the acid from contacting the teeth. (The honey is to help the liver metabolize the salt.) And we rest, preferably lying down. In twenty minutes our energy is better, but we try not to squander this precious commodity. We "take it easy." Our foods are fruits (except oranges and grapefruit which are more alkaline than acid), green vegetable juices and herbal teas. Every hour we take two grams of vitamin C for the rest of that day and the next and when awake at night. Frequently we press the tongue against the slight bump, "button," in the roof of the mouth which stimulates action of the thymus, the gland involved with energy production and the immune system, and tap the breast bone three inches below the collar bone two or three times. (That's over the thymus, to stimulate it.) Another way to restore energy: with thumb and finger, squeeze each side of the fingers of the other hand at the base of the fingernail, seven times for women, nine times for men. Notice the changes in color from pink-red to white as you do this. Squeeze all fingers, and toes if possible. This stimulates circulation at turnaround points. Another thing to do to get much needed extra oxygen into the system is to do deep breathing as you rest. If it's cold outside do not open the window near you. Rest and drink juices, and give thanks to God for the healing He is doing.

COLD SORES: see HERPES, SIMPLEX.

COLIC: acute abdominal pain caused by spasm, a paroxysm or twisting.

In babies or adults, colic usually means a potassium deficiency. Most Americans are deficient in this mineral to some degree because so much of it is lost in food processing or poured down the sink when the water of cooked vegetables is drained off. Such a practice contributes to heart failure, for not only lack of potassium but magnesium and other minerals necessary to heart health are lost.

According to Adelle Davis and her extensive research into medical journals, one gram of potassium chloride given by injection to colicky babies can quickly relieve them. Our nutritionist doctor had mothers measure one gram (a scant one fourth teaspoon) into a small dish and sprinkle a tiny bit of it in baby's water, food and milk over a twenty-four hour period. He said those mothers reported the end of colic in a day or two. He had them continue with the dosage for a few days then reduce it to one eighth teaspoon for a few months.

To rectify a potassium deficiency (and colic), one can take potassium chloride dissolved in water, juice or milk. For near fatal potassium deficiency after taking diuretics and other medications that further lowered the serum level that caused severe and prolonged vomiting and diarrhea, Elizabeth was given ten grams of potassium (chelated) a day, tapered off in a couple of days to five grams, then maintained for several more days, and finally tapered down to two or three grams a day. For years after that almost fatal potassium deficiency experience, she had to take from one to three, 250 milligram tablets in addition to her high potassium diet of fruits such as cantaloupe, bananas, and dark green leafy vegetables that include lambs-quarter and dandelion, the plants highest in potassium. On those rare occasions when her potassium was low she suffered colic just like a baby.

COLITIS: spastic or inflamed colon.

Problems of the colon are so common today they almost seem the rule rather than the exception. Many things, singly or in combination, can cause colitis. It should be determined before an effective nutrition plan can be devised. Often that cause is poorly digested carbohydrates as, for example, cooked cereals and baked products. When this is the case, digestive enzymes may be helpful. Yogurt, kefir or acidophilus cultures may help restore the beneficial bacteria to the intestines. Colitis may also result from food allergies, in which case the Kinesiology or muscle test (see appendix, Kinesiology Testing), may be used to determine the offending food.

Most of us over thirty-five have heard a doctor say that one bowel movement every two or three days is natural and not harmful for some people. Their textbooks usually stress *regularity* instead of frequency. This is proving to be very wrong. Doctors are estimated to be high in the ranks of constipated people. They say this is so because they are too busy to heed the call of nature for themselves and put it off, thus causing the feces to become impacted and allowing toxins to be reabsorbed into the bloodstream. The incidence of colon cancer among them is high. Doctors are reported as having the shortest life span of any of the professions.

Once in awhile colitis, brought on by a combination of stress and food allergy, flares and we immediately go on our colitis regimen. It consists of daily enemas followed by wheat grass juice implants (see Appendix: Wheat Grass Implant), a mild stimulant containing potassium. We also juice fast for four days. We then return to a more normal diet of raw, pureed fresh green leafy vegetables (comfrey and dandelion are the best), raw pureed root vegetables and fresh fruits, yogurt or kefir and raw, sprouted cereal grains and other sprouts.

For Elizabeth there are musts: avoidance of cooked whole grain cereals; avoidance of meats; avoidance of overeating; thorough mastication and salivation; eating sprouted seeds, papaya, banana and olive oil. (see also CANDIDA ALBICANS INFECTION)

CONJUNCTIVITIS: an inflammation and abnormal thickening of the mucous membranes lining the eyelids and covering the white part of the eye.

Such symptoms as pus, redness, itching and swelling may occur and may be caused by deficiencies, allergies, virus or bacteria, or by chemical irritation, dust or smoke. As in most eye diseases, such nutrients as vitamins C, A, E and B2 are especially needed.

A lovely friend of ours in her late twenties whom we have known since her girlhood, came to visit after a few years of absence. She was suffering from such severe conjunctivitis that it was threatening degeneration to the optic nerve. The doctor treating her eyes had not been able to help her. We studied all we could find on the nutritional approach to recovery. After discussing it with us at length and realizing the harm her eating of much pork could be doing, she chose the following program: an all-natural mostly raw diet; primary yeast—three tablespoons a day with meals; eight grams of vitamin C, taken in one gram doses around the clock; vitamin B2, five milligrams; vitamin B6, five milligrams; vitamin E, 800 IU. Two years later when we visited her and her husband and two small children in their home in Mexico, her eyes were almost normal. Only the conjunctiva in the corners of the eyes remained a tiny bit thick. There was no inflammation, no itching, burning, blinking or white matter. A happier, more grateful young woman we have never seen.

CONSTIPATION: a disorder of decreased motility of the muscles of the large intestine.

Constipation is unknown in agricultural areas of the world where few or no processed foods are available and a high residue diet is eaten. In our own country it afflicts more than half the people, many of them children. It may result from food allergies, lack of exercise, being too busy to heed the call of nature, regular use of laxatives, too much animal protein, daily worries, overrefined foods such as sugar and white flour, liver dysfunction or mineral and vitamin deficiencies—especially magnesium and potassium for motility, vitamin C, and inosital, a B vitamin.

Constipation is a disorder in which the decreased motility of the large bowel allows too much water to be reabsorbed, leaving the stool too dry and firm (impacted)—and difficult to expel. It may result from a variety of other causes: continued use of drugs; inadequate bile flow that allows undigested fats to react to iron and/or calcium to form hard soaps; hypothyroidism; prolonged nervousness, and grief. Constipation, according to internal medical physicians, is the beginning of degenerative disease. Most of the foods of a conventional diet lack sufficient fiber, are sticky and adhere to the intestinal walls, causing poor absorption. It usually indicates the first stage of an unhealthy bowel. In such a condition ingested nutrients cannot be properly utilized. There is poor absorption into the blood stream which means insufficient nourishment for the cells and the body suffers malnutrition. Without enough substances for maintenance and repair, the body begins to age prematurely. And premature aging, the beginning of body breakdown, inexorably and subtly erodes to degenerative disease.

To permanently correct constipation, these causes must be eliminated. The Kinesiological or muscle test (see Appendix, Kinesiology Testing) for allergies can indicate what foods, drugs and synthetic and natural supplements one might be allergic to. Remember, no matter how good or how nutritious a food might be, if you are sensitive to it, that food is bad for you. It weakens the body and adds to the toxins the intestines may already be loaded with and having difficulty expelling. For many years leading up to the time Elizabeth's skin and colon cancers were diagnosed, constipation plagued her. After she got on an all-raw diet to battle cancer, constipation, although relieved somewhat, was still a problem. The all-raw diet, adhered to 100 percent, agreed with her 100 percent except for constipation. Elizabeth tried several colon cleansing programs consisting of the use of herbs with psyllium husks (hull) or flaxseed and got fair results. Even then she had to resort to enemas frequently. She thought, "If the diet is sufficiently bulky from my much enjoyed fresh fruits, vegetables, sprouts of seeds, legumes, cereal grains, soaked nuts and dried fruit treats, then there must be something wrong with the motility of the intestines." For good motility the muscles of the intestines need potassium for contracting and magnesium for relaxing. Her excellent diet was replete with potassium and magnesium, yet maybe not enough for *her*. We were in Mexico where we couldn't buy potassium chloride, but we could buy magnesium, not tablets, but plain, unflavored milk of magnesia. Elizabeth started with a teaspoon of it in water before breakfast, lunch and bedtime. The very next day she had better elimination and the day following, three good, normal bowel movements. That is just right, for we eat three meals a day of approximately the same size.

Bowel movements should be twice or three times daily. The feces should be soft, at least an inch in diameter, somewhat dark, fairly smooth, and float briefly in the water of the toilet before they slowly settle. If the feces is yellow it indicates a liver dysfunction. If frothy and foamy, pancreatic dysfunction. If odorous, it indicates putrefaction. Meat and animal products eaters have putrefactive bowel movements. Defecation should be an easy flow without having to strain. There should be little or no need for toilet tissue, just as wild, healthy animals need none.

Since we eat natural, mostly raw foods and Elizabeth takes a little extra magnesium, we have no constipation problem. People often ask us about wheat bran. Frankly, we hesitate to suggest wheat bran. It is too harsh for many. It is an incomplete fiber. It does not absorb water. Oat bran is far superior, has all essential fibers, is not harsh and is higher in nutrients. Sprouted cereal grains—wheat, rye, oats, barley—and sprouted (hulled) buckwheat provide excellent fiber along with super nutrients like abundant B vitamins, minerals and vitamins A, E, K and C in food yeast and in spirulina plankton. Despite this wonderful diet, some people still have a sluggish colon, indicating a possible need for extra magnesium and sometimes extra potassium. There are good liquid calcium-magnesium preparations for helping move the feces down and out painlessly. A newer supplement, magnesium citrate, which is readily assimilated, is also now available. Potassium chloride tablets or chelated potassium help with the natural function of the bowel in addition to the magnesium.

For the family we occasionally make granola bars with bran. But bran is high in phytate which binds the utilization of zinc and iron in the body. When people eat an all natural diet, they naturally get enough fiber. There is no need to eat bran which is nonabsorbable and irritating to the bowel.

We both have our regimen of exercises. Elton prefers morning exercising. Elizabeth prefers taking the strenuous ones in the morning, but doing yoga exercises before retiring. In addition we walk at least two miles a day, five days a week. How great we feel!

CRACKED LIPS: chapped, burning lips.

Dry, chapped or cracked lips result from a B vitamin shortage in the early stages. If the diet is not corrected soon the cracks become sore and painful and appear at the corners of the mouth, around the base of the nose and at the corners of the eyes, along with watering of the eyes. This condition, with our optimal diet, occurs only when we are under undue pressure as when our beloved sons and families all come and we are ten members to be fed, entertained and housed for a few days, and we neglect to take yeast and/or spirulina plankton for extra vitamin B complex needed. The miserable burning, cracking dryness quickly disappears when we take two tablespoons of the yeast and one half teaspoon spirulina plankton. Especially vitamins B2 and B6 are needed. The amount of these two vitamins found in foods is small but primary yeast and spirulina plankton supply it abundantly. A great temptation is to take the synthetic vitamins in tablet form. It's so easy. But most people actually are allergic to the synthetics. Some have found if they take yeast and/or spirulina plankton, then add the specific vitamins in small amounts (bits broken off the tablets), they can benefit. Their distressing lip symptoms disappear in a day or two.

In children and most fairly healthy adults, we have found that once an all-natural diet that includes all kinds of sprouts that are replete with vitamins is undertaken, all B vitamin deficiency symptoms disappear like morning dew in warm sun—steadily, pleasantly.

DANDRUFF: white scaling of the scalp.

One member of our family controlled dandruff with sulphur soap shampoo, another with a vinegar rinse after shampooing. Still another by rubbing castor oil on the scalp a half hour after shampooing. All during college and years after, dandruff showed up periodically on Elizabeth's scalp. When she got off table sugar and onto an all-natural diet it completely disappeared. Table sugar and B vitamin deficiency go hand in hand and the two together may be the greatest cause of dandruff. Many therapists say stress is a major cause. Yet what is wrong with the body that can't cope with the stresses encountered in a busy life of hard work and the setbacks we must expect? It is more often junk food, manufactured beverages, too much coffee, tea, alcohol, etc. In other words, faulty and deficient nutrition allow our bodies to fall prey to any and all diseases. In a nutshell, for eliminating dandruff: an adequate, all-natural diet, acid shampoo and/or vinegar rinse.

DELIRIUM TREMENS (dts): violent tremors induced by excessive prolonged use of alcohol, also said to be brought on by loss of trace minerals and calcium.

The late Dr. William A. Ellis told us that by giving trace minerals and calcium with some magnesium, he had stopped many a case of delirium tremens during his forty-two years of practice.

A person suffering from delirium tremens is woefully lacking in most every nutrient known, especially magnesium and vitamin C. The man we helped was eager to supply the missing magnesium, which soon stopped them. He readily launched into the nutrition regimen we tailor-made for him after his doctor pointed out his many other deficiencies.

DIABETES: a disease that impairs the ability of the body to use sugar and causes sugar to appear abnormally in the urine.

Diabetes is the so-called "prosperity" disease principally caused by consistent overeating of especially refined carbohydrates (white flour products, sugar, animal proteins and fats). These are converted to calories when eaten in excess and laid on as avoirdupois—body fat—unless burnt off by extra exercise. Five out of six diabetics are overweight before diagnosis of this disease which is unknown in countries where the poor never have enough to overeat.

Emphasis for the diabetic should be on raw vegetables, fruits, sprouted seeds and legumes, soaked nuts and cultured milk products like yogurt, if tolerated. *Raw foods stimulate the pancreas and increase insulin production.*

Diabetics need carbohydrates, the natural, unrefined, slow digesting ones. Oats, millet and buckwheat are wise choices. Fruits are a good source of carbohydrates. Fresh fruits contain fructose, a natural sugar which does not require insulin for its utilization. Bananas, apples, avocados and grapefruit are especially good. Green beans and Jerusalem artichokes are excellent. Although this artichoke is classified as a starchy vegetable, it contains considerably less starch than potato. Garlic, too, has been found to reduce the blood sugar of diabetics. Aside from the restricted diet and exercise, strict avoidance of overeating is imperative. Sugar, white flour, alcohol and salt are to be avoided.

Sufficient minerals are very important for control of diabetes. These include magnesium (for avoiding constipation), calcium and the trace minerals chromium and manganese. Diabetes is more prevalent in rainwater and soft water areas. Diabetics and people who wish to avoid diabetes might do well to drink hard mineralized water.

According to the late Dr. Frederick R. Klenner, ten grams daily of vitamin C (taken in at least five doses) helps diabetics heal wounds normally.

There are health institutes like Hippocrates in Boston and The Health Institute of San Diego in Lemon Grove, California where diabetics go and learn to eat, exercise and to better understand the nature and healing of their disease. Those who follow the guidelines to natural living enjoy improvement. A goodly number find their doctors can reduce or stop their intake of insulin. And some experience the miracle of healing completely.

DIAPER RASH: an inflammation or "breaking out" of the skin under the diaper of an infant.

Some infants are sensitive to the soaps or detergents used in washing diapers. Usually the rash will disappear when the diapers are washed with pure soap, rinsed four or more times, and line dried. Sometimes a rash appears on the diaper area of a baby because that may be the tenderest spot. Finding and eliminating the infants's allergy to food or washing powder by surrogate testing (see Appendix: Children's Kinesiology Testing) that family adults can do, can end the problem.

According to a Canadian study, diaper rash on babies wearing disposable diapers is three times as prevalent as on cloth diapered babies. The polyethylene and polyester coverings of disposable diapers—both toxic, nonbreathing, petroleum products—keep baby's skin hot (103 to 104 degrees) and produce a damp, moist hothouse for bacteria to grow in.

Disposables diapers are not only a health hazard, they are an expensive luxury. They cost eight and one-half percent more than diaper service, and nearly twice as much as home machine washed and line dried diapers!

Besides being health suppressing, disposable diapers may well be a health problem to everyone since there is no "proper" way to dispose of them. Thrown in the garbage that ends in land fills, they harbor bacteria that can be carried by rain washing through the land fill or by rodents to water supplies, homes and pets. According to national park authorities, disposable diapers comprise a shocking litter problem, second only to beverage containers.

Citizens of at least two states, Oregon and Washington, have introduced legislation to outlaw the use of disposable diapers in their states. Supporters of these bills contend industry lobbyists killed both initiatives. The town of Torrington, Connecticut banned disposable diapers.

Wrote one young mother, "Elizabeth, can you do anything about the use of disposables, so bad for our babies? Most young mothers don't have any idea how dangerous they are." We were happy to give her the name and address of a young organization called HEALTHIER CHILDREN/HAPPIER FUTURES (see Directory of Products, Sources & Services).

DIARRHEA: loose or liquid bowel.

Metabolic diarrhea may result from digestive and absorption problems, biochemical imbalance, or severe deficiencies of the B vitamins and minerals. Or it may be the body's way of kicking out some food or combination of foods that cannot be properly digested. In such a case one should be thankful for this marvelous ability of the body to take care of a problem that has unwittingly developed.

If diarrhea persists for more than a couple of days, you may want to do something about it. Here are some things that work for many of us who have had the problem. Eat only cooked rice and applesauce made from fresh apples until diarrhea stops. They should be small frequent meals and you should chew each bite at least forty times. After diarrhea has stopped, take sprouted cereal grains such as oats, millet and buckwheat, preferably eaten raw; teas made from carob, sweetened with honey; dried blueberry tea; primary yeast and/or spirulina plankton for the B vitamins and minerals; potassium chloride, one to two grams, and magnesium chloride or magnesium citrate, 600 to 1,000 milligrams.

The parasitic diarrhea Elizabeth had in Sri Lanka (Ceylon) years ago, was cured after a Singhalese dentist, much interested in nutrition, put her on a very nourishing diet. Here it is: white rice and unsweetened applesauce for three days; then raw applesauce made in blender, or apples chewed extremely well, and brown rice. As condition improves, millet; hull-less, raw buckwheat ; oats (whole grain) ideally sprouted and eaten raw; raw fruits and vegetables; bananas and papaya are especially good (these fruits along with cultured milk as kefir, yogurt and buttermilk should be given to infants). All during treatment and recovery period, take four to eight cups of herbal tea— cinnamon, carob and blueberry are best, essence of peppermint and amaranth; kelp, one half teaspoon, and one tablespoon yeast with meals; betaine hydrochloride, two to three tablets after meals.

Elizabeth's recovery was swift. In just three weeks, she was able to climb Sigeria Rock, a mountain-size rock the shape of a barrel stood on end, a feat for anyone.

We have found betaine hydrochloride tablets are the best insurance against "turista" in topical countries. They are available in health food stores. Two taken during or after a meal have none of the adverse reactions of often prescribed Entero-vioform. Incidentally, it has been banned in most countries because it is so toxic.

DIZZINESS: a whirling sensation in the head with a tendency to fall; vertigo or Meniere's disease.

Many people accept dizziness as a part of some illness they are suffering. And it may be. Yet dizziness has many causes— injury to or infection in the inner ear, psychological or severe physical stress, low blood sugar, lack of oxygen in the blood, low or high blood pressure, brain tumor, stroke or anemia, all of which are quite readily diagnosed by a physician. An oftentimes overlooked but increasingly frequent cause is nutritional deficiency. Elizabeth was relieved of Meniere's disease after taking brewer's yeast (one tablespoon with meals), with an additional ten milligrams a day of vitamin B6 and pantothenic acid and salty foods (for adrenal exhaustion). Elton's dizziness disappeared after taking brewer's yeast, twenty-five milligrams of niacin in the form of niacinamide, and manganese, a mineral indicated in problems of balance.

DREAMS: a series of thoughts, images or emotions occurring during sleep.

Bad dreams and nightmares frequently occur to hypoglycemic sufferers after eating sugar or some allergen-bearing food at night. When the blood sugar is maintained at a normal level, dreams are good. When it is extremely low, nightmares often occur. When the blood sugar level is not quite sufficient, dreams may be no more than tense or disturbing.

Traumatic experiences of children can cause bad dreams and nightmares but they are found to go hand in hand with low blood sugar, both as a result of the trauma and a processed junk food diet full of sugar. By correcting the diet, you can change the dream scene to one of pleasantness.

One member of our family for years could not recall his dreams. Since his zinc deficiency was recognized, then corrected, he vividly recalls his dreams. The inability to recall dreams or recall them clearly is a symptom of zinc deficiency.

DRUG ALLERGY: altered body reaction to drugs.

Physicians are finding an increasing number of their patients allergic not only to prescription drugs, but to chemical additives in foods and supplements and in ointments and cosmetics. When one reads of the adverse effects of drugs listed in the *Physician's Desk Reference,* one wonders how anybody can take any kind of drug, the side effects are so numerous and serious. Some of us are extremely sensitive to drugs and chemicals. *The best drugs for us are those left bottled and sitting on the drug store shelves.*

If inadvertently one encounters a chemical in something, or has to take a drug, such as Novocaine at the dentist's or aspirin for a headache or sinus neuritis attack, he or she may find the adverse reaction is greatly lessened if two to four grams of vitamin C are taken with the drug. Vitamin C is, among other things, a powerful detoxifier.

DRY MOUTH: xerostomia, lack of saliva, cotton-mouth.

Although dry mouth is related to age, it is not an inevitable part of aging. People in greater numbers than you may think experience this annoying problem. There are many causes and fortunately many things we can do to eliminate them. Dry mouth is a common side effect of drugs, especially mood altering ones such as antidepressants and antipsychotics. Antihistamines can cause dry mouth as can drugs used to treat Parkinson's disease and stomach problems. Potassium deficiency is also a common cause.

Dry mouth may be a common allergic reaction to foods, fabrics, building materials, chemicals, treated water, sprays, paints, etc. The list seems endless. Polyester and formaldehyde in buildings, and commonly used to keep fish fresh, cause a growing number of people to have xerostomia.

Among other causes are anxiety, stage fright, sudden injury and bad breathing habits. Radiation therapy usually severely and *permanently* lowers the salivary function.

Many of us have experienced dry mouth occasionally for some of the above reasons or simply because we do not drink enough water. When the cause is removed, the symptom usually disappears.

Yet another cause of mouth dryness experienced by an estimated million Americans is Sjogren's syndrome or dryness syndrome. In this case the autoimmune system overworks, causing the body to react against itself. This was one of Elizabeth's problems when discharged from the hospital with "near hopeless" gastroenteritis. After the fasting experience in another hospital, finding what foods gave her no adverse reaction, and getting on an all-natural diet that she could eat, she had no more dry mouth.

After we designed a similar nutritious diet of foods for an elderly lady with painfully dry mouth, her mouth was so much less dry and she felt so much better that she went off the "heart calming drug," to quote her. Another couple of days and her mouth was "nice and moist."

Many people have reported to us their recovery from dry mouth after they greatly improved their diet. Some have reported relief after taking vitamins A and C, plus potassium.

DYSLEXIA: see AUTISM.

EAR PROBLEMS: hard ear wax, partial deafness, noises, fluid in the ear.

A number of ear problems, as too much hard wax, can be prevented if the diet contains sufficient vitamin A (its precursor is carotene) found in dark green leafy vegetables, and bright yellow-orange vegetables and fruits. For us that is not less than 25,000 IU a day of the vitamin A precursor. Our almost daily eight ounces of green drink with carrot (juiced together) alone gives us 25,000 to 50,000 IU of carotene.

One member of our family who neglects ingesting sufficient vitamin A softens the wax in his ears with a drop or two of sweet oil (obtainable at drug stores) in the ears. For a few more days he uses a glycerin drop or two, then douches the ears with warm water. The softened wax washes out quite easily.

Elizabeth's hearing was restored from partial deafness, caused by aspirin taken for the pain of sinus neuritis, after her nutrition was vastly improved and supplemented with the B vitamins, vitamins A and E, brewer's yeast, rice polish, and juices of dark green orange vegetables.

A member of our family has less deafness since correcting low serum iodine and also cholesterol deposits by taking a tablespoon of lecithin granules, six tablets of kelp a day and maintaining a diet of all natural foods with no sugar or white flour.

Noises in the ears (continuous ringing, roaring, hissing, whirring, known as tinnitus) may have many causes. It could be a result of high blood pressure, drugs, low blood iodine, neuritis or inflammation of the nerves, or cholesterol deposits in the arteries. Problems in the small intestine, constipation and colitis can also cause ringing, roaring, or hissing in the ears. Improving the function of the intestines, overcoming constipation (see CONSTIPATION) and vigorous physical activity out of doors can lessen greatly the ear noises that are so annoying.

"Fluid in the ear" concerns pediatricians today much as did large tonsils and adenoids of a generation or two ago. An operation called tympanostomy in which a plastic tube is placed through the eardrums, performed on millions of children a year in the United States, has replaced the million-plus tonsillectomies that used to be performed at a staggering cost. Yet tympanostomy was introduced on the basis of theory alone.

Studies have shown, in the case of a tube being inserted in only one ear, the other serving as a control, there resulted little difference in the ears. No demonstrable benefit was evident in the tubed ear which, incidentally, had scar damage and permanent perforation.

Research and experience show this kind of middle ear infection to be self-limiting, a condition which is not improved by any of the current methods of medical treatment, says Dr. Robert S. Mendelsohn, world recognized pediatrician, writer and lecturer. To tonsillectomies and adenoidectomies are added tympanostomies as surgical operations to be mostly avoided in favor of the healing methods of time and good nutrition.

EDEMA: an abnormal accumulation of fluid in connective tissues.

Water retention, or edema, is so prevalent that it is often not considered as remarkable, especially in children where it is frequently overlooked. Many people have lived with slight edema for so long they think the bags under their eyes and puffy hands and feet are normal for them.

Edema can be caused by heart failure or kidney failure; too much salt; too much ammonia buildup from undigested protein especially animal; food allergy; or other conditions. Whatever the cause, edema means kidney involvement and may indicate adrenal exhaustion.

Vitamin C (eight to fifteen grams a day in spaced doses, as recommended by the late Dr. Frederick R. Klenner) acts as a diuretic for edema. It activates arginase which breaks down the amino acid arginine, resulting in production of urea which is one key to tissue fluid balance.

On the verge of B vitamin and mineral deficiencies, particularly calcium and vitamin D, Elizabeth was subject to edema if she became exhausted, was exposed to too many pollutants or ate cooked foods in restaurants while traveling. Much of the potassium has been lost in such foods and too much salt added, creating an imbalance in the body and causing water to be held in the cells by excess salt. Now that she eats all-raw foods, with an abundance of sprouted seeds, leafy green vegetables, and fruits, seeds and nuts, she has no water retention. And the bouts with kidney problems and bladder infections that made life miserable for her years ago are now a thing of the past. We have found an all-watermelon or an all-grape diet for two or three weeks cleanses out impurities of the system, clears up health problems, makes us look ten years younger and gives us such energy we feel like we're floating when we walk.

EMOTIONAL DISTURBANCES: see AUTISM.

EMPHYSEMA: a disease of swelling that destroys the small air sacs of the lungs.

These sacs become stretched and then lose their elasticity and allow air to accumulate in the lungs. This condition progressively decreases the ability to utilize fresh air. Repeated bouts of respiratory diseases, cigarette smoking, dust, chronic asthma, and bronchitis may lead to emphysema with wheezing, difficulty in breathing, and shortness of breath resulting.

Although no member of our family has had emphysema, we know lots of people suffering from the disease. Elizabeth used to experience the panic of fighting for enough oxygen to breath in smog filled cities, especially when coupled with high altitude as in Mexico City. In that altitude there is thirty per cent less oxygen than at sea level. When air pollution is high there can be as much as twenty per cent less. That adds up to fifty percent less oxygen than clean sea level air. We have found that endurance to such exposure is much greater if we take fifteen to twenty grams of vitamin C. Vitamin C is a remarkable oxygen conserver and detoxifier in the body.

Recently new friends, a charming active couple, came to us to learn what might be an effective diet for emphysema. At this writing he is so much better they have canceled their rather purposeless retirement plans and are launching into a new career in philanthropy. Here is what happened. We muscle tested them for food and substance allergies and found many, which they immediately eliminated. Because the man needs all the oxygen he can get for comfortable living and lung recuperation, he chose to eat only live foods which have all their precious oxygen, and to take green vegetable drinks that include comfrey, dandelion, and carrots that help keep oxygen in the cells. He also does deep breathing exercises several times a day and takes long daily walks. They live on a hill in Portland away from downtown traffic. Their often washed air is quite good.

Again, let us say that an all-natural, preferably raw diet gives optimal nutrition for healing the body of whatever disease. Supplements to meet deficiency needs, however, have been found to be vitamin A (50,000 units), vitamin B complex, folic acid, pangamic acid (fifty milligrams three times a day), vitamin C (eight to twelve grams a day), vitamin D, vitamin E (1,600 to 2,000 IU per day), and easily digested, complete, mostly vegetable protein for maintenance and repair of the lungs. (see also SMOKING)

ENERGY PROBLEMS: lack of energy, fatigue, exhaustion or lethargy.

Any and all of these can be caused by dozens of ills. Physicians pointed out that the low immune system Elizabeth lived with, anemia, the low blood pressure, allergies, constipation, low blood sugar and the "discouragement" (their diagnosis) she endured left her too weak to function properly. These were the "causes," to quote them.

Yet what prompted these "causes"? In Elizabeth's case, as in many, a low immune system translated to low energy (see IMMUNE SYSTEM). Correcting that over a span of many years has been a contribution to her energy. Maintaining a pH of 5.5 (see Appendix Body pH Chart) greatly contributes to good energy. Discovering her allergies and removing the allergen-bearing substances from her diet and environment was a real boost to the immune system and to energy. Adoption of a maximum, nourishing health program which ended anemia after a deficiency of copper, folic acid and vitamin B12 was corrected by taking spirulina plankton, and the resultant normal blood pressure (formerly very low) have contributed to her energy flow and supply. Daily walks and a half hour of exercises—breathing, sit-ups, isometrics—keep her fit, energetic and praising God for His guiding her through the "valley of the shadow of death."

ENURESIS: see BED-WETTING.

EPILEPSY: a nervous disorder causing convulsions, with symptoms of noise sensitivity, twitching, muscle spasms, irritability, apprehension, tremors and/or bed wetting.

The most exciting things happening in the treatment of epilepsy are nutritional. An extensive study by biochemists and physicians recently revealed that many epileptics are hypoglycemic and allergy-prone.

A nutritionist doctor friend of ours quite emphatically says epilepsy is a classic example of deficiency disease. The critically short supply of vitamin B6 and magnesium, or the body's inability to absorb them, can cause epilepsy in all ages from new born babies to the aged. However, he says panthurenic acid tests show that some people with epilepsy do not have vitamin B6 deficiency, indicating the vitamin has no corrective effect. In such cases, our doctor friend gave them only extra magnesium along with a greatly improved diet with invariably productive results. When he gave patients vitamin B6 (one to five milligrams for babies, five to ten milligrams for children, ten to twenty-five milligrams for adults), magnesium (200 milligrams for babies, 450 milligrams for children, 500 to 800 milligrams for adults) and a diet high in all nutrients, he was able in a day or two to take them off anticonvalescent drugs. Soon all symptoms disappeared, even depression and mental retardation. He enjoyed grateful patients freed from the awful suffering and stigma of epilepsy. Now retired, he's receiving encouragement from us to write a book or at least an article on epilepsy. We cannot help but be extremely impressed by complete nutrition, correct for each individual person, which helps the body right itself from disease.

ESOPHAGUS: see CANDIDA ALBICANS INFECTION.

EXERCISE: regular use of body parts to thwart atrophy and maintain good body tone.

There's a time worn adage in referring to the body: "If you don't use it, you lose it.." While it makes a good catch phrase, it isn't quite true. You don't usually *lose* it, you lose the *use* of it. You can get it back—but that takes a lot of dedication, persistence, self-discipline and hard work. Even so, it's worth it.

How much better to *keep* the use of all our muscles and feel tip-top in the doing! Our bodies were made to be active, to have good circulation, to walk, to sweat, to breath hard now and then, to do vigorous physical work and recreation. Without sufficient exercise the entire system becomes sluggish and nutrients cannot be properly digested and wastes expelled. They may stay in the blood and in essence become minute toxins, the start of degenerative disease. Volumes have been written on the necessity of sufficient, vigorous exercise. They, like volumes on nutrition, need not only to be read, but heeded.

There are exercises for everyone, regardless of disability.

Even a person paralyzed from the neck down can exercise the eye muscles, the jaws, the muscles of the scalp, face and neck, and to sing and yawn to exercise those of the throat and lungs. A paraplegic we're acquainted with does the astronaut's neck exercises and yawning. All shut-ins can be helped by having pointed out to them those parts of the body they can move, and being encouraged and taught to move them with a real purpose, the purpose of exercising for feeling better and possible recovery. Every moveable part of the body should be moved over and over again for maximum health and well-being.

There are exercising gadgets, machines and equipment so numerous we will attempt to make only the most limited comment. Some are therapeutic for some people; and some have only placebo value. But some types of equipment we've found quite helpful. The rebounder, or home trampoline, is excellent for muscle tone, including the heart and for circulation. We wouldn't be without one. After trampolining five or so minutes, a person will test strong Kinesiologically. After jogging, he or she will test weak. For Elizabeth, the backswing is great. It is not at all advised for people with high blood pressure, back injuries, or heart problems. The buyer of *all* exercising equipment should consult experts in the field for guidance before making a decision to purchase. A good idea, before spending all that money, is to try out the exercise item after being advised.

EXHAUSTION: see ENERGY PROBLEMS.

EYES: infections of and other problems as floating black dots, the need to wear dark glasses, etc. (see also GLAUCOMA, CATARACTS, CONJUNCTIVITIS, RETINOSA PIGMENTOSA).

An eminent ophthalmologist friend, the late Dr. Purman Dorman, believed that all diseases of the eye begin with a vitamin C deficiency. Another one says vitamin A deficiency is present in all eye problems. This is not surprising because nature intended for the eye to store vitamin C, yet most people don't take sufficient vitamin C for even minimum daily needs, let alone enough to store. Doctors generally believed that vitamin C was not stored anywhere in the body. This erroneous assumption came about as a result of autopsies that were made on unhealthy bodies. In recent years medical scientists have discovered that normally vitamin C is stored, in the order of concentrations per proportionate organ size, in the adrenal glands, in the eyes and in the pancreas. In addition to vitamin C, vitamins A and B2 are necessary for the health of the eyes.

Bacterial infections of the eye are many, from low grade to severe, such as staphylococcus. Low grade infection and/or body toxicity may be expelled through the ducts of the eye and appear as a thick white substance that temporarily blurs the vision, irritates the lids, causes a slight sticky watering and frequent batting of the eyelids.

Elizabeth has had this condition of the eyes many times after a severe illness as pneumonia, back injury, or mental or emotional stress from one of life's temporary "downs." However, praise God, He revealed how to deal with it. Go on a cleansing diet of any *one* fruit in season (apples, grapes, papaya, watermelon, or, if winter, grapefruit, bananas or dry organic prunes, water reconstituted), and extra vitamin C. At the same time wash the eyes twice daily in sodium ascorbate water.

To do this dissolve one eighth teaspoon sodium ascorbate in one tablespoon lukewarm water. Put in two eyecups or two hospital pill cups. Fit the cups into the eye sockets, tilt back the head and bat the eyelids slowly, allowing the vitamin C solution to bathe the eyes for a count of thirty seconds. Lower head, remove cups, wiping away only the drip of water. Allow the extra moisture to stay until it evaporates. This puts the vitamin C where it is immediately needed. The eyelids and surfaces are not only cleansed, they absorb some of the vitamin C. How rested one feels after an eyebath of vitamin C water!

Severe infections, including staphylococcus, can be cleared up in a few days with *raw, unstrained honey.* Imagine Elizabeth's shock one morning when she awoke with her eyes stuck shut with thick, yellowish matter. Immediately she knew it was staph infection and how it got there. The day before, after irrigating her staph infected sinuses (see SINUS PROBLEMS), she had blown her nose and failed to protect her eyes with a cleaning tissue. This allowed a fine spray of water to hit her eyes and infect them. She was concerned for she knew staph infection can cause blindness. Since our nutritionist physician was away attending an alternate therapy conference, we began to review our resources. We recalled Dr. Jarvis in his book, *Vermont Folk Medicine,* said no bacteria or virus could live in raw, unstrained honey. In another chapter he said cataracts in the early stages could be cured or stopped from progressing by a drop of unstrained honey twice a day in the eyes.

Putting these two vital bits of information together, Elton let fall from a toothpick a drop of honey in each staph infected eye as Elizabeth lay prone. The burning on contact was intense for ten or fifteen seconds. She was soon able to open her eyes and allow the honey-tear solution to bathe the eyes. After a few minutes the burning greatly lessened and the eyes began to have a clean, though sticky, feeling. More tears dissipated the honey and Elizabeth wiped her cheeks, never touching her eyes. In a few more minutes they felt all right and she went about her day as usual.

We repeated the honey treatment morning and night, the infection steadily disappearing. The morning of the third day there was no infection. We were so excited we went to see our physician who had just returned. Always reluctant to use antibiotics and other strong disinfectants, he was delighted to hear what we had done, and the beautiful, swift results. He immediately made notes on how we "stopped the staph," as he said. He put the treatment into his practice after making one noteworthy change. He added a tiny bit of procaine to the raw, unstrained honey to eliminate the pain to the eyes when applied.

An annoying problem is a black spot, or spots, said to be dead, unsloughed cells floating in the peripheral vision. They disappear when B2 is adequate. It works for us every time. After overworking or suffering undue stress, we up our sprouts and primary yeast, the best plant food source of vitamin B2.

All sorts of eye problems in children have been found to respond favorably and quickly to regular exercise on a trampoline or rebounder, a "discovery" made in the 1930's. Many children have been relieved of the crutch of eye glasses after such exercising.

A word about colored or tinted glasses. The custom of wearing tinted and dark glasses is universally accepted as necessary or fashionable. Yet only a few people should wear them except to lessen glare on such occasions as sun on snow, water or white desert sand. A real need for dark glasses is usually a vitamin A deficiency. Dark glasses soon become a "crutch" for the eyes and take away the need for them to exert themselves to adapt to different strengths of light. Looking through pink tinted lenses, so often seen now, weakens a person when tested

Kinesiologically. They shut out strength giving rays of the sun necessary for total health. If people insist on dark glasses, they might choose a type of smoked, full spectrum lens that does not screen out the rays of sunlight God provided for good sight. Neither of us consciously abandoned our various pairs of dark and tinted glasses when we went on an optimal, raw diet. We just naturally wore them less and less. How wonderful to be free of the "crutches," the nuisance, the expense of tinted and dark glasses!

FACIAL SIGNS OF HEALTH PROBLEMS: Blemishes, wrinkles, lines, poor color and texture are some of the telltale conditions denoting condition of health.

Liver and pancreas dysfunction can cause dark spots like enlarged freckles on the face, neck, hands and arms. A sallow or yellow skin color may raise suspicions of a sick liver. An ashy, pasty white skin may spell anemia, cancer or any number of serious metabolic disorders. White spots may indicate vitiligo, a B vitamin deficiency, and dark areas a vitamin C deficiency. Vertical lines between the eyebrows can reflect below normal function of the liver from toxic or malabsorbing intestines and vertical lines in the earlobes are often present in heart trouble patients. "Whistle" marks around the mouth are prone to develop when there's a B vitamin deficiency, a condition occurring more in women than in men. Wrinkles over the face tend to reflect a "similar condition inside," some doctors quite simply state. Dark circles under the eyes may indicate allergy, puffy eyes a kidney problem, and squinting eyes may be indicative of a vitamin A deficiency or nearsightedness. Too much ingested salt, according to experts, may be reflected in a light, whitish blue circle around the outer edge of the iris. And irises that float above the lower lid, exposing the white of the eye—considered to be a "dramatic" look—is often a serious vitamin B6 deficiency. (The Japanese call it *sam paku.*)

Such facial "signs" are numerous indeed. Some people do not believe in them. They are not necessarily "proven." They are observations, interesting to many, both in and out of the healing professions.

FASTING: True fasting is going completely without food or juices for a period of days, taking only pure water.

A "juice" fast, although advisable for some, is not a true fast.

People wishing to fast should seek the counsel of a physician or person experienced in fasting.

Primitive peoples, aborigines, ancient Indian tribes, people of Bible times, and the Chinese of antiquity all knew the effectiveness of fasting for health of body, mind and spirit. Remember that fasting is as natural as rain; as old as mankind. Animals know to fast themselves when they are sick. Jesus said, "When ye fast," not "If ye fast." It was taken for granted that we fast for cleansing, healing and renewing the body for the clear-functioning mind that God intends us to have.

Fasting is a natural way to health. It is necessary for giving our best to God in worship, praise, thanksgiving and knowing His will, for maximum learning leading to the wisdom He wants for us, for a loving nature, and for the patience and calmness so necessary for getting along with others.

Over a period of many years, Dr. Theron Randolph in Zion International Hospital in Chicago developed and practiced diagnostic fasting. The basic principle is quite simple. A patient fasts on pure spring or well water until he or she is well, then is tested on one food every four or five hours. Going through the fast is not simple. Withdrawal from food, alcohol, drugs, tobacco or caffeine puts the patient through misery, pain and sickness. The more severe the illness the more agonizing and the longer is the period of fasting.

Both of us have fasted several times for different reasons and with equally good results. We both encourage people to explore the subject through study and consulting professional therapists who can help them.

Because people often learn from the experience of others, we will tell of Elizabeth's fasting experience. Many years ago the hospital internist and specialist told Elton that Elizabeth had such severe gastroenteritis and related problems there was little hope. He discharged her, he led us to suppose, so she could die at home. Later our nutritionist doctor called to say he thought he had found the answer to the questions Elizabeth's critical condition posed. "I think you should fast. This last week my wife and I stayed in a fasting clinic until we felt well. It took me four days and her five and a half. We're still testing foods every four or five hours and finding we're getting allergic reactions to nearly half of the things we've been eating. I feel sure this is the way for you to get well. You have to fast out all the toxins and impurities so your body can heal itself."

Elizabeth listened, awestruck. Had he lost his marbles? Fasting, she agreed with the conventional doctors she had seen most of her life, was starvation, a sure way to death. However, Dr. Silver's voice was full of such enthusiasm she could not oppose him. In a small voice, Elizabeth told him he'd have to convince them both.

It took a week. Elizabeth had reached a point where her system had all but shut down. She literally could not digest anything. Elton piled her into the back seat of the car next day and drove down the Oregon coast where a young pediatrician-allergist had been given two rooms in a pediatrics wing of the hospital to fast a few patients whose illnesses were too complicated or baffling for orthodox medicine. This pediatrician a few years before had been just such a patient himself when he went through Dr. Randolph's clinic. He was so amazed at the swiftness and sureness of the results that he learned all he could from Dr. Randolph. Returning to his practice, he arranged for his own fasting clinic. Elton checked Elizabeth in, then he checked out the mortuary!

Elizabeth was immediately given an enema and magnesium, potassium and sodium bicarbonate to eliminate as much as possible to shorten the fast. Fresh water was placed on her bedside table along with salt which she was to take in small quantities now and then to keep from dehydrating. For three days she was so miserable she could not visit with Elton, listen to the radio, read or sleep. The morning of the fourth day she awoke from a short, sound sleep feeling great. The doctor came soon after. "You look good," he said, then quickly added, "But we'll wait a few hours to see whether or not you go back into withdrawal." Elizabeth didn't quite know what he meant but by noon she understood. Suddenly, as though she'd been tossed into a pit of misery, she relapsed into withdrawal. For four more days and nights she felt worse than ever. Her body played back every major suffering it had known. Stomach cramps doubled her for an hour, then stopped; restless legs accompanied everything; the agony of postpartum childbirth pains against the Caesarean section for the birth of our first child; an excruciating sinus neuritis, so intolerable off and on years before; the exquisite pain of a severe childhood back injury; the heavy, aching chest of pneumonia, and on and on. Nothing but the restless legs lasted more than an hour or so, fading as something else took its place.

Elton read to her for hours, nutritional and ecological books, papers and articles the doctor brought because we were interested and he wanted to share and compare research information and experience with kindred spirits. Elizabeth's memory of those long days is one of his soothing voice droning on and on through what otherwise would have been an unbearable ordeal. The effort she had to make to listen, to try to be civil, kept her from complaining and feeling sorry for herself. She had to "measure up" for his sake. The eighth day Elizabeth awoke after a deep four-hour sleep, the longest she had had. She felt absolutely wonderful. She had pep and energy. She could clearly read a sign across the street that had been a blur. Her sense of touch was acute. Her hearing was so keen she could listen to the many natural sounds of early morning way in the distance and separate each one from the other. Her nose was like a bloodhound's. What a marvelous set of sensations! What joy they were!

In minutes the doctor came. "You look great." Elizabeth told him she felt super. "We'll wait until night before we test you with a food. We must make sure you are through withdrawal. You really feel good?" She assured him she'd never experienced such a feeling of well being, then added she felt very near to her Maker.

"We all do after we've fasted out the impurities, the toxins in our bodies so that we are well."

What a day it was! We chatted with such enthusiasm we were like newlyweds. Life was suddenly sweeter than it had ever been. After hovering near death, then achieving great health, Elizabeth felt renewed not only physically but mentally, emotionally and spiritually. She thought she knew the joy of the Lord and all his goodness to us, but nothing quite compared with this experience.

In the two weeks that followed, testing one single natural food every four or five hours, we found, of the thirty-six served her, Elizabeth could eat only eleven. Twenty-five gave her an adverse reaction. Those twenty-five had been causing most if not all her illnesses! It was incredible. She could not believe it. But it was true.

The symptoms after eating something wrong for her ranged from merely annoying to severely painful, according to the diary she was required by the doctor to keep. For instance, peas caused the little blisters on her throat and tongue that had been so puzzling from time to time. Broccoli gave her diarrhea. She was deathly sick with vomiting after eating fresh caught red snapper. Naturally raised beef, chicken and turkey caused stomach cramps, sick headache and trapped gas, in that order. Potatoes caused impacted bowel; wheat caused severe exhaustion. An hour after eating she crumpled to the floor. The doctor ordered an immediate blood test which revealed a sugar level of 42. On a previous normal morning after no reaction to food the night before, the fasting level was 80.

Other things tested, as several vegetables steamed briefly, blurred her vision, gave her watery eyes, stiff neck, dizziness, a feeling she had been drugged. Oranges in a few minutes caused sharp pains in her stomach and the intense pain of arthritis she had been increasingly suffering. Mango fruit gave an itching, burning rash on her face, beets made her hoarse, and uncolored cheddar cheese produced copious amounts of sinus discharge. But the worst reaction of all was from a baked potato. From her bilateral hernia, through the stomach, into the small intestine, it caused havoc. She had eaten it at six o'clock, her next-to-the-last evening in the hospital and gone to sleep soon after. She awoke from a nightmare at midnight, consumed by nausea, cramps and migraine headache. Such diarrhea followed she thought she would expire. Her eye and face twitched with the earlier diagnosed tic douloureux and lower back syndrome pain struck again.

When Elizabeth ate a food that caused problems, the doctor gave her the following remedy to rid her system harmlessly as quickly as possible: milk of magnesia, two tablespoons; two rounded teaspoons of a mix of one part potassium bicarbonate and two parts sodium bicarbonate, dissolved in a glass of water and drunk soon after the allergic reaction appeared.

It usually took four to six hours to flush out her system so she could test another food. Her appetite returned soon after the "purge," as she called the elimination. Elizabeth left the hospital with eleven foods she could eat. Twenty-five had made her sick. She needed twelve in order to have one different food each meal for twelve meals, four days in a row. This is called a four-day rotation diet. At home she tried frozen blueberries. They agreed. As time went on she found more and more foods, particularly the unusual ones, like moose meat, that she could eat. Our nephew went hunting in Canada and got a moose and put it in our deep freeze! Her body had had no chance to build up a sensitivity to such foods. Repeating a food too often, especially an incomplete one such as white flour, sugar, and processed things puts a person in jeopardy of becoming allergic to it. In other words, it takes away energy rather than giving it. Food should always give energy. And energy she had at long last. How wonderful! And how marvelous to be able to eat and thoroughly enjoy foods that gave *no* problems. God had kept His promise to renew her youth like the eagle's. Psalms: 103–5

To have firsthand experience, Elton water fasted for five days. The first three days he felt unwell, especially the third day. However, he puttered at some carpentry work around our place, muddling through, as he says. The fourth and fifth days he felt fine and late the night of the fifth day went off the fast by eating half an apple chewed extremely well. He favors fasting for many people. Since her hospital fast Elizabeth has fasted three times until well: a juice fast for six and one half days after two years of fighting colon cancer which resulted in her expelling the old dead tumor from her lower bowel (see "Our Personal Stories"); once for seven days to get over the excruciating pain after a meninges sheath injury in the lower back, and once for nine and one half days of water fasting only a year before this writing to get over severe bronchial pneumonia (see PNEU-MONIA). Elizabeth loses just under a pound a day, Elton just over a pound a day. At 107 and 170 pounds we carry no extra weight.

We suggest a water fast for health restoration, maintenance and recuperation—but only after a physician has examined the patient and approved either a water fast or a juice fast. And we strongly recommend a step-by-step study on fasting in *How to Get Well* by Paavo Airola, and *Fasting* by Paul Bragg or any book or article on fasting your nutritionist physician recommends. Personally, we feel the chapter on juice fasting in *How To Get Well* is among the best. When we juice fast, it is the one we follow.

From our own experiences with fasting, here are a few do's and don't's:

Do
* Fast during a quiet, few days interval; drink pure water as desired, with a bit of salt now and then. Rest often. Break the fast with only a little food at a time, like fruit or juice, first fruit then vegetable.

Don't
* Take strenuous exercise. Fast more than four days without a doctor's supervision. Break the fast with animal protein. Tell everyone you're fasting. Take vitamin and/or mineral supplements when you fast.

Note: Soon after the start of a water fast, the body pH will be somewhere between 5.0 and 6.0. Both of us have found invariably our body pH is 5.0 to 5.5 when we fast. When not fasting we feel the best when our pH is that reading on the nitrozene paper. Many people cleanse their bodies well on a juice fast of one to two weeks. However, for the allergy-prone person, this may not be good because of possible allergies to some or many of the juices.

The very ill person should fast in a hospital under the constant supervision of trained professionals.

Remember that fasting is as natural as rain; as old as mankind. Animals know how to fast themselves well when they are sick. Should we know less?

FATIGUE: see ENERGY PROBLEMS.

FEVER: the elevation of body temperature above normal.

While it varies from individual to individual, the body temperature usually ranges between 97 degrees to 99 degrees Fahrenheit. Fever may be a warning sign that something is wrong. It accompanies many diseases, the majority of which can readily be diagnosed. It is nature's way of "burning up" bacteria and virus.

FEVER BLISTERS: herpes simplex, lip blisters or fever blisters which occur when the resistance is low.

Lowered resistance signals the need for extra nutrients, especially the B vitamins, vitamin C and the amino acid lycine. When we are threatened with fever blisters as a result of colds, flu, fever or extra stress, we take extra amounts of these vitamins. At the first sign of the tingling, burning on the lip which is the beginning of a blister, we rub it with apple cider vinegar or a drop of oil, then dry vitamin C powder. The oil helps the vitamin C to stick. In twenty to thirty minutes the tingling is gone and the blister stopped. Fever blisters occur when the body pH is high (alkaline). We take extra vitamin C, apple cider vinegar, lycine and betaine hydrochloride. As a result we seldom have fever blisters. (see also HERPES, SIMPLEX)

FINGERNAIL PROBLEMS: fingernail abnormalities that reveal much about the health of the body.

Pink smooth-surfaced, gently rounded, strong, rapid-growing fingernals indicate good health and an adequate diet. Abnormalities of the fingernails invariably indicate inadequate nutrition. When processed foods are avoided and the diet is maximum, fingernails become strong, problem-free and fast-growing. Infections around nails can be cleared in a few days by applying vitamins C and E topically or taking daily doses orally.

Here are a few abnormal conditions and what symptoms they may indicate:

Split, brittle, extremely thin nails are usually a sign of nervousness, lack of protein and/or vitamin A.

Slow growing nails often denote general bad health, drug ingestion, the stress of cold, inadequate diet and potassium deficiency.

Longitudinal (length) ridges mean anemia or cobalamin (B12) deficiency.

Transverse (width) ridges signify menstruation problems, deficiency of vitamin B6, and pantothenic acid may be indicated.

Longitudinal cracks may show unbalanced diet or B2 deficiency.

No Moons area a sign of vitamin C deficiency.

Nails tending to curve down over end of finger indicate essential hypertension.

Nails growing away from quick at corners and sides are caused by a fungus from B vitamin deficiency.

Cloudy white across the center or white spots suggest a zinc deficiency.

Hangnails imply protein, vitamin B and/or folic acid deficiencies.

FLATULENCE (gas): the presence of an excessive amount of gas in the stomach and intestines.

From what we read and hear in lectures and in conversation with physicians, biochemists, nutritionists and therapists, we are led to believe there are about as many causes for flatulence, singly or in combination, as there are flatulence sufferers. However, from our long trying experience with the problem, and the experiences of countless others—the problem seems to affect well over fifty percent of people over forty-five—we believe there are three major causes: food allergies, lack of stomach acid, and overeating. For years, doctors told Elizabeth the gas she lived with was caused by undigested foods. True. But what caused them *not* to be digested? With both of us, not enough hydrochloric acid (stomach acid) was definitely at least one cause. Elton takes two betaine hydrochloride tablets after each meal, Elizabeth takes three to four, depending on the size of the meal and amount of protein in it. Even with that, we can get gas by doing several things: eating too fast which means air is swallowed; not enough chewing for good stomach digestion; eating something we are allergic to; too much cooked starch (Elizabeth hasn't eaten anything cooked for years and rarely has gas) and synthetic vitamins that most people's systems cannot properly take care of. Other causes could be medications; megadoses of vitamin C to ward off a cold, flu or bronchitis; constipation; carbonated soft drinks; caffeine (in coffee, bakery goods, tea and soft drinks); diuretic; not enough alkalinity in the small intestines for the pancreatic enzymes to be utilized in digesting the food (see bibliography, *Brain Allergy* by Dr. William Philpott); liver and gall bladder trouble (lack of bile); nervous upset just before, during or after a meal, especially dinner; too much white sugar; and overeating.

The above are *some* of the causes. Let us repeat the four main treatment modalities that have helped so many people diminish or get rid of flatulence. They are, 1) finding the food allergies that you and a responsible adult can test for by Kinesiology, then eliminating totally that food; 2) lack of stomach acid. Ask your physician for the test. It's quick, simple, inexpensive, painless. Just a pill to swallow and a urine sample afterwards tells the story; 3) overeating and 4) potent, synthetic vitamins.

FLUORIDE: see CHLORINE and TOOTH PROBLEMS.

FLUORESCENT LIGHTS AND PROBLEMS THEY CAUSE:
poor vision, headache, dizziness, a feeling of unreality, etc.

Before we civilized ourselves into semi-invalidism, we got an abundance of natural light by being outdoors. Light from ordinary fluorescent and incandescent bulbs does not provide us with the full spectrum light the sun gives off. Plants, animals and humans living mostly in such light do not have the vigor and health they have under natural light.

Fluorescent light is worse than ordinary incandescent light. This light leaves out so much of the natural light that students attending classes illuminated with it have a shorter attention span, become irritable, sluggish and tired. Factory, plant and office workers do not perform as well. Many cannot function normally, some have eye or balance problems, or severe headaches, psychological and emotional problems, feel "spaced-out," or suffer intense fatigue.

Some animals are unable to reproduce while living mostly under fluorescent light. They became healthier, were not quarrelsome, reproduced and lived longer when the light was changed to full spectrum.

Full spectrum lights are made to emit the full spectrum of rays the sun gives off. Where installed, factory, office, and plant employees are healthier and perform better with no strange and subtle health blocks slowing them down in thought and action. Dr. John Ott, the Disney photographer, ex-banker and scientist who developed this health-giving light, has also developed a full spectrum, heavy plastic window glass, eye glasses and contact lens. Our ophthalmologist friend says eyes especially suffer unless they get plenty of natural light. With no glasses or with full spectrum lenses, fluorescent lights and window panes, eyes do get enough natural light. Outdoors we get total electro-magnetic spectrum from cosmic rays, gamma rays, X-rays, ultraviolet, infrared, radio waves; our brief exposure to outdoors does not make up for what we receive behind glass "filters." (Read: *Health and Light* by Dr. John N. Ott)

Here are a few examples of the harmful effect the common fluorescent and incandescent light has on most forms of life including man. Many research animals living under daylight white fluorescent light were completely bald. When natural light is inadequate, we are malilluminated. Ninety-eight percent of the civilized world suffers from malillumination, says Dr. Ott.; Modern glass lets in most of the visible light but only one percent of the total light from the sun, experts tell us.

FOLIC ACID DEFICIENCY: a need or lack of this part of the B vitamin complex which functions as a coenzyme, with vitamin B12 and C, in breaking down and utilizing proteins.

Many people today have anemia and poor meat and animal protein digestion because of the overlooked nutrient folic acid (folacin). This may result in water retention from the ammonia from those undigested proteins so often overlooked in patients suffering edema. If salt restriction doesn't end edema, ask your doctor to test you for ammonia build up from undigested protein.

Without sufficient folic acid the following problems may show up: decrease or loss of appetite; faulty utilization of sugar and amino acids; cell division and healing slowed down or stopped; hair, eyebrows, eyelashes fall out; recovery from anemia slowed or prevented; burning lips and sore mouth; hair growth and color subnormal; lack of a feeling of well-being.

About the time Elizabeth learned that she had a severe folic acid deficiency the FDA prohibited the over-the-counter sale of folic acid except in minute amounts of .01 milligrams. In order to get plenty of the all-important vitamin she either eats two cups a day of a raw green leafy vegetable pureed in a blender with one and one fourth cups water, or drinks a glass of juice made from mostly green leafy vegetables. When she neglects ingesting this much for even a few days she still experiences burning lips although with no decrease in appetite and lack of the exuberant feeling of well-being unless the neglect is prolonged.

Folic acid deficiency plays a significant role in preaging, memory failure and many other problems. It is found in abundance in green leafy vegetables.

FOOD ADDITIVES: chemicals, foreign to the body, used in foods to preserve, color, flavor, emulsify, moisturize, extend shelf life, bleach, etc. The Food and Drug Administration (FDA) allows nearly 1,000 additives for food and lists another 4,000 as *probably* safe. The average person on a conventional diet ingests five pounds of chemicals a year. That's five pounds of toxins. Poisons! They make the body like a stagnant pool instead of the clear, rushing, energy-filled stream God intended. Trash foods are full of additives; overheated oils robbed of their original nutrition through processing; sugar loaded or artificially sweetened; overcooked or irradiated with microwaves. Bit by bit, health is destroyed as surely as letting a toxic chemical slowly drip on a plant.

The most devastating result is what is happening to our children. Rare is the completely healthy child, and common now is the slow learner, the mentally retarded, the birth defect child. As research and clinical studies are made, it is becoming clear that most of these problems result from malnutrition, many times accompanied by alcoholism, smoking, street drugs, prescribed drugs and food additives.

The answer seems too simple for most to heed—good, natural nutrition through predominantly living foods. Most of our adult population has health so impaired by a bad conventional diet they may never know good health again. The children's scene is even more gloomy. Many, by continuing with the highly processed, artificial, nutrition-robbed diet TV advertising promotes, haven't a chance for good health.

FOOT PROBLEMS: burning and/or painful feet, a condition resulting from fatty deposits plugging the small arteries in the feet, decreasing their supply of oxygen.

This is yet another manifestation of vitamin deficiency, especially B6, C and E. In Elizabeth's case, burning feet followed any unusually stressful occurrence such as pneumonia, prolonged overwork like the last few weeks of meeting a publication deadline, massive exposure to environmental toxins or trauma from the loss of a loved one. All these things make greater demands on the B vitamins than Elizabeth can supply. For her, the best thing to do is take extra brewer's yeast, spirulina plankton and sprouts of all kinds, as the Biblical Daniel ate for the excellent health he maintained until his death.

GALLSTONES: balls or "stones" which mainly consist of cholesterol but sometimes of bile pigments.

Gallstones form in the gallbladder when there isn't enough of the right kind of fats and sufficient vitamins E and A. They can be dissolved by eating all natural foods including unprocessed fats and taking extra vitamins A and E.

A middle aged man angrily opposing gallbladder surgery for gallstones that his doctors and family insisted on, called us and said he would do exactly as we suggested if we could outline a nutrition program that might help him. We did. (His telephone bill must have been astronomical for he was 3,000 miles away.) Months later he dropped us a card to say no more gallbladder attacks, no more stones, but he had had to rent a beach cottage for two months to be away from his family to eat right. They no longer think him crazy, however.

GANGRENE: blood poisoning caused by bacteria that has poisoned (contaminated) the blood.

Gangrene is being cured by intravenous vitamin C (sodium ascorbate) in amounts of forty to 180 grams in a twenty-four period for a few days. Vitamin C is a powerful infection fighter. Gangrenous sores are quickly healed when sugar is poured in them and dressed two or three times a day. Honey will do the same. So treated, the wounds are easily, painlessly dressed. Several doctors in America and Europe are using this age old remedy, which leaves few or no scars.

GAS: see FLATULENCE.

GLAUCOMA: tension in the eye that can cause pain, burning, blindness and detached retina.

Glaucoma does not need to happen. It can be stopped from progressing and even be reversed. Many years ago two ophthalmoligists at the University of Rome, Italy, medical school developed a formula for treatment after learning of Dr. Frederick R. Klenner's research and clinical results with massive doses of vitamin C. Drs. Virno and Vietti found that vitamin C given for glaucoma, the amount gauged by the weight of the patient, could accomplish recovery in the early stages of the disease, and improvement in even advanced cases, reported Dr. Frederick Klenner in 1967. (see "Our Personal Stories")

GOITER: enlargement of the thyroid gland.

Despite iodized salt, goiter is still not unusual. As a result of woefully inadequate nutrition when in college, Elizabeth developed goiter which was treated off and on through the years by Lugols solution (iodine) and thyroid tablets. The results were questionable. But since her vastly improved nutrition regimen, supplemented with kelp for minerals, her thyroid functions consistently better. We believe that the massage of this neck gland and the exercises developed for the astronauts which we learned some years ago (see appendix: Exercises for Astronauts), also help keep the thyroid gland functioning.

GOUT: pain caused by uric acid, needlelike crystals in the soft tissues around the joints, usually the toes, fingers and knees.

Possibly the only consolation for gout is the high uric acid in the blood that goes along with high I.Q. However, there is relief for gout—a vegetarian diet with no animal proteins and other high purine foods that cause uric acid crystals.

Can anything be done for painful gout besides drugs that rarely work? How joyous to report there is! Acupuncture helps to relieve the pain. Fruits, vegetables, sprouted seeds and legumes, soaked nuts, and if lactose is tolerated, yogurt or kefir, preferably made from goat's milk, help to relieve the cause. Another possibility is the diet for arthritis.

Here is the list of no-no's: meat and wheat products (raw sprouted wheat is well tolerated). Fats cooked at high temperature. In high temperature frying or broiling, fat goes through a brief rancid stage; if it is used repeatedly, the rancidity increases and the fat, like tar or rubber, soon becomes completely indigestible. This is one of the two greatest single causes of artery plaque and fatlike sludge; the other is hydrogenated margarine and oils which have little or nothing of the original nutrition. Other no-nos are animal product foods, refined sugar, and citrus fruit.

Sour cherries help many rid themselves of the excruciating pain of gout. Years ago gout in Elton's right hand helped to make life miserable for him until he learned about cherries which relieved the pain considerably but not entirely. When he gradually adopted an all-raw diet the gout finally disappeared. A few winters ago in Mexico where the citrus harvest was especially good, he bought a twenty-five pound sack of tangerines. For three days he ate between twelve and twenty tangerines a day! The morning of the fourth day he awoke with his big toe throbbing so badly he yelled as he stood up. It was red and so swollen he could not wear any kind of shoe. So terrible was the pain that he reluctantly consented to see the acupuncturist the next day. After the treatment the pain was so much diminished Elton could smile. Next day he had another treatment which ended the pain and swelling in a few hours.

One more time Elton had gout flare up when on a trip. He drank our hosts' tall glass of fresh-squeezed orange juice. The attack this time was in the opposite toe and in the right hand. Two trips to the acupuncturist and most of the pain was gone. After a week, all sign of gout had faded. That was three years ago. No more than twice a week Elton may eat citrus fruit and then only a bit of lemon juice on a salad or a section or two of orange or grapefruit. (see also JOINT PROBLEMS.)

How thankful we both are to have learned from experience the cause and what helped for the cure so that we can tell others.

GROWTH PROBLEMS: (see ZINC DEFICIENCY).

HAIR ANALYSIS: a reliable test for minerals in the tissues; one of many diagnostic tests. A test often used and considered by many in both orthodox and alternate practice to be reliable, is the hair analysis test for minerals in the tissues. Correlated at the same time with results of a serum (blood) analysis for minerals, it may become a meaningful diagnostic procedure.

A tablespoon of hair is taken from the base of the lower back of the head. Only hair growing from next to the head to an inch and a half out is used. The determination of minerals contained in this most recent growth of the hair is made by a nuclear spectroscopy procedure, considered to be a very accurate analysis. Not only amounts of all known minerals, but balances and/or imbalances in them is revealed. For instance, the ratio between sodium, and potassium, magnesium and calcium, iron and copper, etc., can be determined. From these test results, correlated at the same time with a blood test for minerals, physicians and therapists of other disciplines can pinpoint deficiencies and imbalances of a patient and determine what supplements may be needed for optimal nutrition and eventual health.

HAIR PROBLEMS: dull, slow growth, falling hair.

The following hair problems we have helped through special nutrition. To combat falling hair you can eat a completely adequate diet with extra folic acid, biotin, inositol and B6, pantothenic acid and PABA (Para Amino Benzoic Acid). Thinning hair indicates a lack of amino acids as found in yeast, folic acid, rich green leafy vegetables and spirulina plankton. For graying hair we take pantothenic acid, folic acid, PABA and copper. Elizabeth's hair is now mostly dark and Elton's is far less gray than most people his age. The Cherokee Indian remedy for baldness: "In spring cut small notch in wild grapevine. Catch juice. Several times a week rub into scalp. Some men have restored hair. The remedy also *keeps* hair on the head." Compliments of Elizabeth's Cherokee great grandmother.

HALITOSIS: bad breath.

Halitosis can come from diseased tonsils or gums. More often it is from faulty digestion and constipation. Bacteria multiply fantastically on the undigested food in the intestines, releasing putrefactive gas and causing accompanying foul breath and/or coated tongue.

Eating all natural foods, mostly raw, taking yogurt, kefir, acidophilus milk or culture and high vitamin B6 foods (bananas, rice polish and bran, egg yolks, green leafy vegetables, etc.) can rectify the condition.

A peculiar offensive breath odor is common among many older people and some not so old. It usually indicates a lack of hydrochloric acid and may be easily rectified by taking betaine hydrochloride or glutamic acid hydrochloride, found at health food stores.

HANGNAILS see FINGERNAIL PROBLEMS.

HAY FEVER: allergic rhinitis, a reaction of mucous-bearing membranes of the nose, eyes, bronchi and lungs to dust, animal hair, feathers, pollen, foods, etc.

Symptoms include watery, itchy eyes and nose, sneezing and irritability. Stress situations and alcohol can also bring on an attack of hay fever.

The obvious way to treat hay fever effectively is to remove the irritants. Since that is not always possible, treatments have been developed to help the sufferer. Vitamins A, C, B complex, plenty of dark green leafy vegetables for minerals, particularly magnesium, potassium and calcium, bee pollen and raw, unstrained honey all help.

There are a number of folk remedies that work for lots of people. We list here some of those that people we know have found to be effective. Take two teaspoons daily of raw, unstrained honey produced in your locality six weeks before the start of the hay fever season. The pollen in the honey acts as an inoculation. When the pollen starts and hits your nose, your body thus may be able to cope with it. Take it through the season. When our second son got through the high school and college experience of junk food and ate a more natural diet of vegetables, fruits, nuts and sprouts and took extra vitamins C and A, his hay fever became minimal. Elizabeth's own severe hay fever reaction to pollen, dust and other irritants has rarely occurred since she adopted an optimal raw diet, adhered to at home or away. We thank God daily for this hard earned lesson.

HEADACHE: pain, either in one spot or all over the head, neck and shoulders.

A spot pain can be caused by an allergy, neuralgia or neuritis, as sinus neuritis. Pain in and around the eyes and temples is often a sign of eye problems, a top-of-the-head pain oftentimes is caused by overeating and/or indigestion; a base-of-the-head pain by nervous tension or tension from over work and sore muscles of the neck and shoulders. A severe all-over-the-head or migraine headache may be brought on by hypoglycemia (low blood sugar) and/or severe allergies. A dull, all-over headache can be caused by polluted air, lack of sleep, or anxiety. A constant headache might be from worn-off teeth which let the jaws come too close together, from ill-fitting dentures, from mandibular (jaw) problems, or from constipation of long duration.

We only touch on some of the main causes of headaches. As one physician friend working in conjunction with a chiropractor-acupressurist says, there are about as many different causes for headaches as there are people suffering from them.

If the cause is one or more of the above-mentioned ones, then it stands to reason the cure is the removal of the cause! Many causes such as overeating or eating too late at night can easily be removed. Exercising the neck and shoulders (see Appendix, *Exercises of the Astronauts*) or a long, brisk walk in clean air frequently brings relief.

In the case of persistent headache, a nutrition-practicing physician should be consulted. High blood pressure can cause such a headache. Or you may find relief at the hands of a naturopath, an acupressurist, an acupuncturist, an osteopath or a chiropractor.

When a headache persists or recurs frequently, make every

effort to observe your pattern of living, diet, activities, indulgences and exercises. The analysis will help your therapist find the cause and eliminate it. (See also FLUORESCENT LIGHTS.)

HEART PROBLEMS: any abnormality of the heart, whether congenital or acquired.

The most prevalent problems today are acquired, those occurring from body abuse through malnutrition, lack of exercise, overeating, drugs, alcohol, tobacco, stress, repeated anesthetics, severe environmental pollution, etc.

It has been well established that diet has a lot to do with maintenance of a healthy heart, preventing initial or succeeding heart attacks, and recovery from heart attack. Almost as important as diet is exercise.

Heart attack was first correctly diagnosed in 1893 by a Canadian physician, Sir William Osler. Up until then, and indeed long after—until 1926—doctors continued to call a heart attack "sudden death." It was believed to be a result of severe indigestion. Up until 1949, heart attack was mainly recognized by the patients's acute indigestion and/or angina pectoris, and received little if any help from the family doctor. For the next eighteen or twenty years, when heart attack was caused by "coronary thrombosis," doctors would put patients to bed.

Space here does not permit us to discuss heart problems except in briefest terms. However, we would like to point out two startling historical facts. Before the turn of the century when machine milling discarded wheat germ from flour and hydrogenation of vegetable oils destroyed the "good" in them (linoleic acid, linolenic acid and vitamin E), the typical American diet contained approximately 150 IU of vitamin E. By 1960 that amount had declined precariously to only fifteen IU. Tragically, by 1980, the average diet contained seven and four tenths IUs of vitamin E.

The increase in heart attack has consistently gone up as the amount of ingested vitamin E has gone down. Doesn't it logically follow that from this undisputed correlation we can conclude that an optimal diet not only could, but would, prevent most heart attacks? We all know people who have survived heart attack and by following their doctor's diet and exercise plan often enjoy even better health than before their heart attack because they lose weight, improve digestion and breathing, lower the cholesterol and phospholipid count, increase their energy, sleep better and have a renewed outlook on life. Diet, exercise, determination, and faith are the name of the game in the challenge of heart attack prevention and recovery.

There are a few generally accepted approaches to heart problems. Vitamin C helps lower cholesterol, strengthens, and helps more oxygen to get to the heart. Calcium acts to calm the heart. Magnesium is necessary for relaxing the muscles; potassium for the contraction of muscles (the heart is a large muscle). Vitamin E conserves oxygen for the function of the heart, eliminates much scar tissue and strengthens the heart. A fast heart may mean a heart weak from insufficient, vigorous exercise, a very prevalent condition in today's western world, but getting better with people exercising regularly more the last few years.

The heart attack situation is improving. The incidence of this problem is less in the last five years. It is going down as exercising, losing weight, giving up tobacco, nutrition improvement and faith gain acceptance. In this case, statistics speak as eloquently as double blind studies.

For a healthy heart, think vitamin C (three to ten grams a day with bioflavonoids); vitamin E (400 to 1,200 IU and/or *fresh* raw wheat germ, plenty of raw seeds and nuts); selenium (yeast is a good source); sulfate for removing fatty deposits in the arteries; an all-natural diet, mostly raw.

HEMORRHOIDS OR PILES: a dilation of veins of the rectum caused by pressure on that part and poor circulation; the sagging and folding of anal membrane which often is accompanied by bleeding.

Although straining because of constipation is considered by many to be the prime cause of hemorrhoids, there are several others, such as liver sluggishness or damage, magnesium deficiency, venous stasis (distended veins) and pregnancy.

For recovery, the "bad" must be removed from the diet: sugar, cured meats, artificial flavor and color, plus preservatives and other chemicals. In other words, all processed foods should be avoided. An all natural fare is mostly raw foods, organically grown. It would include fruits, vegetables, sprouted seeds and grains. Nuts soaked in water for four to eight hours are essential. These foods contain vitamins C, E, and K, which help stop bleeding. They are also rich in the B vitamins, vitamin A precursor, carotene, and the bioflavonoids, all indicated in cases of hemorrhoids.

In our experience and in that reported by many others, vitamin B6 (5 to 10 mg) and magnesium citrate or orotate (200 to 400 mg) two to three times a day, have helped relieve and shrink hemorrhoids. This treatment is especially quick and effective when pregnancy is the cause.

There is no need for the "simple surgery" many in conventional medicine advocate. To the patient the operation is major. Recovery takes many weeks. And the anus and rectal walls are left greatly weakened. A fairly new treatment in which a negative galvanic current is painlessly introduced into the affected vein causing it to shrink, is reportedly very successful. For more information, write to Dr. Shefrin, 5240 N. Casa Blanca Road, Paradise Valley, AZ 85283.

HERNIA: a rupture.

According to *Stedman's Medical Dictionary* the protrusion of an organ or part of an organ or other structure through the wall of the cavity normally containing it.

Causes of lower abdominal hernia vary, but heavy lifting wrongly done (putting weight on stomach muscles), and straining when constipated are the most widely recognized causes. Obesity from overeating, jumping down from a height, heavy coughing, and vomiting are additional causes.

Hiatial hernia is considered to be one of the most common gastrointestinal abnormalities in the Western world, and it is one of the most difficult to detect. Physicians often misdiagnose it as heartburn, indigestion, even heart attack.

When the stomach or esophagus is moved from the normal place, we have a hernia. A common cause is the muscles of the diaphragm surrounding the place of connection between stomach and esophagus become flabby and unable to maintain their tightness, allowing the stomach or esophagus to push through until it's out of place.

Recently it has been noted that hernias occur more often in persons with vitamin C and mineral deficiencies, especially potassium. Vitamin C is for strong colligen, the "glue" that holds the cells together. Potassium is for good contraction of muscles. B vitamin deficiencies contribute also, since sufficient amounts of them are necessary for healthy intestines and good absorption of minerals.

Other than surgery, necessary in some cases, there are things we can do for improvement or correction of hernia: a good nutritional program, proper exercise and weight loss in the case of obesity.

Our Dr. Silver who finally diagnosed the hernia that had caused much of Elizabeth's stomach problem, years later commented about her recovery from hiatial hernia, "I've always felt that given the proper chance, the body could right itself from whatever wrong. God created us self-healing. Many of my nonsurgery hernia cases improved. You are one of two who became symptom—and hernia—free."

How did her healing come about? Elizabeth asked God to guide her in doing the things she needed to do for healing her body in such a way it would *stay* healed. She had finally realized that her *conventional diet* was what had made her a walking medical dictionary of illnesses since she was neither overweight, depressed nor negligent of exercise. Bad diet was mainly the cause. When she went first to an all-natural, mostly raw diet, she began steadily to improve. When cancer of the colon was finally discovered, Elizabeth adopted a completely raw diet. It took years to overcome all her diseases. But through countless trials and errors and incalculable suffering, she grew in the Lord and came to know the security of His love and the joy that knows no human understanding. Elizabeth says "God had a purpose in allowing me to go through more than seventy-five health problems. I humbly, radiantly thank Him for it all."

There is something else we learned from our nutritionist doctor. For a hiatial hernia, lie flat on your back, force all the air out of the lungs while pushing down on the hernia with the fingers of both hands. Use force as you push this spot down, then hold as you inhale a few times. Release and rest a few minutes. He suggested doing this treatment one to three times a day.

HERPES, GENITAL: a virus (herpes genetalia) of the penis or vulva, visibly manifesting itself in small, burning, itching, painful blisters that when broken can cause sores which are difficult to heal.

It is said by some, both here and in Australia, that genital herpes can be overcome by an all-raw diet of organically grown, chemically-free foods, all kinds of sprouted seeds and grains, and natural foods containing a high concentration of nutrients—such as spirulina plankton, brewer's yeast, oat and rice bran. Also helpful are megadoses of vitamin C, exercising in clean, fresh air, plus plenty of rest and faith!

HERPES SIMPLEX: water blisters, cold sores, fever blisters.

Caused by a virus infection and appearing inside or around the mouth and/or on face, hands, lips, genitals and stomach. They occur when the body's resistance is low.

By rubbing on dry vitamin C crystals at the first hint of fever blisters (a tingling, slightly burning sensation) they can be warded off. A little vegetable or facial oil rubbed on the affected spot helps the vitamin C crystals stick to the skin. Repeat the procedure at two to three hour intervals for a couple more times.

Zinc applied topically prevents herpes virus replication (dissolve a fifteen milligram tablet in a tablespoon of lukewarm water and rub on affected area.)

Recent research has shown fever blisters appear when the amino acid lycine is in short supply or there is an imbalance with too much arginine. Chocolate is high in arginine. Eating too much may contribute to the incidence of fever blisters. When these two amino acids are balanced by reducing the ingestion of arginine or increasing the intake of lycine, along with sufficient vitamins C, A, E, and B6 in the diet, fever blisters usually do not appear. Taking apple cider vinegar, by helping to keep the body on the acid side, is good insurance against herpes. (See also FEVER BLISTERS.)

HERPES, ZOSTER: shingles, a viral infection of the nerve endings of the skin.

Itching, burning blisters with crust formation appear on the skin. Neuralgic pain all along the affected nerves is severe and may last for several weeks. The most commonly affected areas are the chest, abdomen or the area just below the ribcage across the back.

Since herpes zoster is a viral disease, megadoses of vitamin C are indicated along with the B vitamins which are necessary for healthy nerve function and vitamins A and E for skin function and healing respectively.

Elizabeth was never more surprised than when she awoke one morning with neuralgic pain from her shoulder down to the hand and little red itching blisters twisting down the arm into the palm. None of our family or close friends had ever had shingles and it never entered her mind that she would have it. But recalling happenings of the day before, we could see some reason for her predicament. We had carried numerous boxes to the garage packed for our new condominium in Mexico. Just as we finished and were nearly exhausted a man we knew came by and out of the blue bawled her out unmercifully. At first she was merely dumbfounded, but later grew furious at the unjustified treatment. (Soon after, he was found to be deeply paranoid from severe food allergy.) The straining of arm and shoulder muscles, fatigue and the emotional upset simultaneously set her up for what happened.

Our nutritionist doctor was away but we called him by phone, explained what had happened and her miserable symptoms. He chuckled, "Sounds like you *do* have a case of shingles." He encouraged Elizabeth to eat all raw foods, up the intake of vitamin C, primary yeast and bee pollen for the B vitamins, and her daily glass of green vegetable juice which she had begun to neglect now and again. Then he said, "Don't forget to rub the blisters often with apple cider vinegar."

The last, seemingly insignificant instruction we forgot until the middle of the day when the summer heat bore down and the burning and itching of the blisters became almost unbearable. When we applied the vinegar the burning and itching completely stopped. The arm felt fine except for the deep, haunting ache of neuralgia. But when the vinegar evaporated, back came the awful burn and itch. Elizabeth decided the trick was to *keep* the arm moist with vinegar.

In minutes she had stripped an old sheet, saturated long bandages of it with vinegar and had Elton wind them around her arm from the shoulder to the most painful blisters of all, those in the palm of her hand. Then Elton put her arm in a long, plastic salmon fish bag to keep the bandage moist, gave her two grams of vitamin C and three teaspoons of vinegar (served with a straw to keep the acid off the teeth), and tucked her in bed for a nap.

For two more days and nights we carried on the treatment, the raw diet, the extra food supplements. The morning of the fourth day Elizabeth awoke early. To our delight, the blisters were gone and so was the redness. No more itching and burning. The neuralgia was still with her but the pain was dull and not difficult to live with. In five more days it completely disappeared. Nine days for conquering a miserable virus. Our nutritionist physician was elated when he called the tenth day to see what had happened while he was gone. On hearing, he exclaimed, "I'm sure that's a record for shingles. Let me jot down a few notes while I have you on the phone."

HIATIAL HERNIA: see HERNIA.

HYDROCHLORIC ACID DEFICIENCY: hypochlorhydria; not enough stomach acid to digest proteins.

Normally, chewing foods generates the enzyme ptyalin in the mouth which in turn stimulates the production of hydrochloric acid in the stomach. But today with the soft, smooth, fiber-poor, processed foods and meat, people chew very little. This slowdown in the stomach's production of hydrochloric acid began in the 1920's when processed foods came into general use. According to experts, by the time people reach age forty in today's world, hydrochloric acid production is slowed to between twenty-five and fifty percent. By age sixty, production of this acid is twenty-five percent to none at all.

Sufficient hydrochloric acid is necessary not only for good digestion, (it breaks protein down to amino acids) but for keeping the pH slightly on the acid side (see Appendix, Body pH Chart) to help protect the body from bacteria and viral proliferation. A physician friend says in his practice of forty years he found that all sick patients, including those with arthritis, cancer and inflammatory diseases, had low or no hydrochloric acid in their stomachs.

The problem is easily dealt with. Because hydrochloric acid is an essential nutrient, it can be bought at health food stores as hydrochloric acid, glutamic acid hydrochloride or betaine hydrochloride. Your doctor can test for your stomach acid level and tell you whether or not you need the supplement and how much to take.

With insufficient hydrochloric acid in the stomach, foods are only partly digested. In the intestines they then are partially absorbed. This means the system is undernourished and loaded with toxins from undigested, fermented, putrefactive foods in the poorly functioning intestines—a perfect setup for any and all kinds of disease. This is why many physicians say all degenerative diseases start in the colon, the cesspool of the body.

HYPERACTIVITY: supercharged, nervous action; abnormally high, sometimes erratic behavior.

Other noted symptoms of hyperactivity are short attention span, lack of concentration, tiredness, irritability, confusion, antisocial behavior, headaches, poor memory, failure to pay attention, and a host of physical problems. Experts—researchers, physicians, biochemists—agree that sugar, caffeine in cola drinks, other refined carbohydrates such as white rice and white flour products, cause hyperactivity. It is what keeps children from learning and adults from performing well in their work and being calm in their homes. There is a direct correlation between hyperactivity in a family and the eating of sugars, caffeine in cola drinks and processed foods loaded with artificial color and flavor and other additives. The number of chemical additives in foods has gone to well over 2,000. Americans now consume an average of five pounds of chemicals in their food a year.

When hyperactive school children were taken off all processed foods and given all natural foods, their behavior changed in a matter of a few days. They became calm, their attention span increased, their learning disability ceased to exist, they had good memory and were agreeable and cooperative.

Despite all the documented evidence of such physicians as Paul Dunn, M.D. and pediatrician in Illinois, and Sidney Walker, M.D.M. and neuropsychiastrist in California, who have done studies on children with learning disabilities and behavioral problems such as temper tantrums, depression and blood sugar disorders, many people do not believe this.

We can only say, if your child or a family member is uptight, quick-tempered, subject to mood swings, emotional, has easily hurt feelings, is impatient, quarrelsome and over active at times, tired and lethargic at other times, take all sugar out of the diet. Drink pure fruit juice instead of soft drinks. Eliminate *all* colas and fruit "drinks." Don't buy any junk foods: prepared, packaged, or processed items. It isn't easy, but it can be done. It saves you money. Our book *Bandwagon to Health* will help you make the change, a change that will make a world of difference in your life. The book was written for people like you. God bless you! Now we'd like to share the story of some friends from Australia.

Two Hyperactive Children Returned to Calm Behavior and Scholastic Achievement by Max Gray, Coff's Harbor, Australia.

Before our third little girl had leukemia and recovered from it, our family went through other drastic health problems. Just prior to starting our family, I was sprayed completely with DDT, a near fatal accident. It took a lot of trials and errors to find out how not only to save my life, (doctors didn't know what to do for me) but regain a semblance of normal health. All natural foods and twenty to forty grams (20,000 to 40,000 milligrams) of vitamin C a day in one to two hour spaced doses finally restored me to a normally functioning person again.

In the meantime our first child, Debbie, was born on November 25, 1967. From the first she was hyperactive. How much the DDT poisoning I got just before she was conceived, and the fact that I was a three month premature baby (preemies are hyperactive prone), had to do with her problem, we do not know.

Debbie slept little and was so active, irritable, and moody we thought we'd go insane. Doctors said we were bad parents and were the cause of her problems. One of the main causes, we later learned, was the family TV, only six inches (though the wall) from the head of her bed.

Our second child, Sonia, born September 7, 1970, was the one who had leukemia.

On September 4, 1973, our third child, Joanne, was born a placid, healthy baby. However, by age two she developed a taste for lollies, ice cream paddles and other junk food, all of which contained sugar and artificial color and flavoring. The family TV contributed its share of the hyperactivity. When a local butcher gave her a party savoloy (a highly "treated" sausage) she became so hyperactive for the next six hours, she threw tantrum after tantrum. It took two days for her to return to normal.

In the meantime, I had heard of Dr. Feingold and his getting to the causes of hyperactivity. Also, how junk foods put a terrible strain on the liver, our detoxifying organ. I also learned hypoglycemia goes hand in hand with hyperactivity, as does, strangely, high intelligence in the affected children. And I heard about A/G-PRO, a supplemental formula of amino acids and minerals. I also learned of an Australian product called Phosco, a phosphorus containing calcium phosphate, sixteen milligrams; iron, eight milligrams; potassium, sixteen milligrams; magnesium, sixteen milligrams. These are called mood minerals. After taking them our hyperactive Debbie and Joanne were in a good mood in a matter of minutes. We were astonished. Along with the amino acid mineral formula, we had two well-behaved little girls who soon became socially popular and achievers in school. Debbie, our eldest, would never have been able to attend high school without our discovering the nutritional-supplemental way.

Note: Elizabeth and Elton again visited these friends of many years while on a speaking tour of Australia during October and November of 1985. They were a beautiful, healthy family, the three girls now well-adjusted, successful young ladies.

HYPERTENSION: high blood pressure.

This condition has been described as the body's corrective effort and defense against certain diseases. It is the result of the body's trying to cope with such conditions as subnormal kidney function, too much salt, degenerative changes in arteries, obesity, toxemia, potassium deficiency, glandular malfunction, or emotional stress from such factors as job pressure, overwork, worry and anxiety. Symptoms may be absent. Or they may be insomnia, blurred vision, dizziness, edema, nervousness, nosebleed, shortness of breath, to mention some.

Whatever the cause, high blood pressure patients must examine their diet. We *are* what we eat and assimilate, and hypertensives we've known who have changed their diet to an all-natural one have without exception lowered their blood pressure. Even if the cause of the high pressure is mainly driving themselves too hard, or other types of emotional stress they haven't been able to change, their blood pressure has lowered somewhat. Those who can eliminate some or all of the cause found their blood pressure lowered to high normal or normal.

As with most degenerative diseases, supplying the body with optimal nutrition means eventual healing because the body has all the building materials for repairing the damage caused by deficiencies.

Emphasis should be on a diet low in sodium and sufficient in potassium for allowing the body to rid itself of retained water. Foods excellent for that are fruits, vegetables (raw), sprouted legumes, buckwheat and cereal grains, soaked nuts and cooked cereals like millet, oats and brown rice. (Garlic, if tolerated, and buckwheat are both rich in rutin, a nutrient especially good for hypertension. Vitamin C and calcium also help to lower hypertension.) Exercise, as usual, is extremely important—walking, swimming, golfing, bicycling, trampolining, etc.

Elton has had mild hypertension most of his adult life. After he quit eating processed foods, sugar, meat, white flour and too

much salt and adhered to an exercise program which includes
calisthenics, rebounding and rapidly walking, his blood pressure
has normalized.

HYPOGLYCEMIA: low blood sugar, the term used to denote
a condition of abnormally low glucose (sugar) in the blood.

It is mainly caused by too much sugar in the diet, liver
malfunction that interferes with release and storage of sugar, or
tumors in the pancreas causing overproduction of insulin. Too
much ingested, refined carbohydrate (sugar, white flour products and with some people, dried fruits) causes a rapid rise in
blood sugar levels, exciting the pancreas to produce an excess of
insulin. This overage of insulin then takes too much sugar from
the blood, leaving an abnormally low level. The process causes
high to low swings in energy known as the yo-yo energy effect.

Symptoms of hypoglycemia (which itself is a symptom)
range from the following: fatigue; weak, restless legs; migraine;
hunger; eyeache; night sweats; nervousness; irritability; edema;
pains in any part of the body; depression and strange behavior
that may be taken for mental disorders. (see appendix, Hypoglycemia Symptoms)

In the 1970's, doctors ordered the glucose tolerance test for
such symptoms, a test that verified the amount of sugar in the
blood at a given time. Then when hypoglycemia was recognized
as a serious and rampant problem among Americans, they
advocated a high animal protein diet low in carbohydrates and
moderate in fats. But time and much experience with increasing
numbers of hypoglycemics soon proved the fallacy of this
practice. Often, it replaced several symptoms with a number of
new ones.

It was discovered that food sensitivities and allergies trigger
hypoglycemia. Each patient's diet must be tailored to his or her
own needs. We are all different. "What is one man's meat
(substance) is another man's poison," said Hippocrates, the
father of medicine who lived between 300 and 400 years before
Christ.

The task of finding those allergies and sensitivities in
hypoglycemia patients has become easier, faster, much less
expensive and more accurate since Kinesiological (muscle)
Testing was "discovered" and developed. While orthodox
physicians remain cool to the test, dentists, chiropractors,
naturopaths, alternate therapy physicians and the nutrition

minded public use the test to eliminate those foods and substances (petrochemical products) that can cause a wide and bizarre variety of reactions. As a result of eating only foods that *give* energy, people are recovering from the myriad, baffling, stressful symptoms of low blood sugar almost as soon as the allergen causing food and substances are eliminated. Tea, coffee, decaffeinate, alcohol, tobacco and drugs should be avoided.

When Elizabeth suffered severe hypoglycemia in the 1960's and was sent to three psychiatrists (the last one recognized the problems she had as physical instead of mental/emotional), we could find no help. There is good help today but not in many places. We feel strongly led to assist others who suffer equally for there is a quick, painless way out: Kinesiological Testing for allergies and sensitivities. For a full explanation, read *Your Body Doesn't Lie,* by John Diamond, M.D., an utterly fascinating little book. It will explain muscle testing of many things and help you to health and energy. When you discover what foods you are sensitive to and eliminate them, then concentrate on balancing the essential nutrients (foods) that give you energy, you'll be amazed at the miracle worked in your life. (See appendix, Hypoglycemia Symptoms.)

HYPOCHLORHYDRIA: see HYDROCLORIC ACID DEFICIENCY.

IMMUNE SYSTEM: various organs of the body that work together to protect and heal it; the defense system against disease and injury.

We don't believe it's necessary for most of us to understand the intricate biochemistry of the immune system. To date, the experts agree the field has only had the surface scratched in study and research. However, experts also recognize that nutrition comes first, such as vitamin A (natural tocopherol), selenium (100 to 500 micrograms), zinc, copper (care should be taken in determining the correct amount *if* a supplement is needed, as determined by a doctor well versed in nutrition), manganese, beta carotene, magnesium/calcium in balance, and potassium/sodium in balance, the building blocks of restored health.

It is a long hard battle in reconstruction. Elizabeth has been fighting it for many years since being given Chloromycetin, a 1950's "miracle" drug, for pneumonia. Eventually it was mostly banned. One of its remarkable side effects was partial destruction of the bone marrow, our white blood cell manufacturing center. In the several years Chloromycetin was given, many recipients of it died later as a result of virus and bacterial infections because their bodies had little or no defense against them. The flu, pneumonia, bronchitis, and severe cold attacks Elizabeth had through the years, each followed by low grade fever, brought her health to a near "fatal" state several times. It took years of faith, persistence, optimal nutrition through all-natural raw foods, and natural supplements to go from twenty percent of normal white (leukocyte) count of the blood to low normal. Somehow the last few years she was able to gain on it, even though each winter she fell prey to bronchial pneumonia because of a chronic bronchitis she hadn't been able to overcome. We heard lectures and read research papers on live cell therapy. A year ago Elizabeth had live cell therapy for bone marrow and has gotten through the first winter in twenty-five years with no respiratory disease. Praise the Lord!

INDIGESTION: see STOMACH PROBLEMS.

INFECTION: contamination of cells by invading bacteria or virus.

Infections mostly occur when the body's defenses are low. To avoid infections we must keep the body healthy with good, natural nutrition. The subject of infection is so vast and can include any and all parts of the body, inside and out, it cannot be discussed but minutely in our limited space. We just want to bring to light a few ages old, very effective treatments for skin and open sore infections.

Table sugar packed into an open sore one or two times a day for a few days ends the infection with no pain, no distress of bandaging (it doesn't stick) and practically no scars.

Egg white, because it contains no iron, upon which bacteria feed, spread over an infection a time or two a day will soon starve the bacteria, thus ending the infection. Run clear, cool water over the sore to wash off, allow it to dry, then apply fresh egg white again. This method has been used since Shakespeare's time.

Raw honey covering the sore and lightly bandaged is also effective. It needs to be repeated twice a day until healed. Bacteria cannot live in honey or sugar. These two sweets dehydrate the bacteria and they die quickly.

INFERTILITY: inability to conceive or to cause conception.

Mostly we are consulted for planning an optimal diet by women after they have become pregnant. Rarely has anyone asked how the *mother and father-to-be* should eat before conception. This is sad, for a good strong sperm and a healthy egg are of utmost importance for an offspring to enjoy radiant, vigorous health. We can readily agree with professionals practicing the natural ways, that much of infertility results from malnourishment.

Infertility has many causes: (1) the tubes may be blocked by mucous preventing the passage of the egg to unite with the sperm. (By a change to natural foods with many fresh, raw fruits and vegetables, regular exercise, relaxation, and sunbathing daily, the problem can be overcome.) (2) poor health of either the male or female; (3) out of position pelvis and spine which may be corrected by manipulation; (4) sterility from taking the pill; (5) orchitis (inflammation of the testicles) in men or boys, with antibiotics given, may later be the cause of malfunction or suppression of the sperm. According to a double certificated nurse we know in Australia, some cases have been corrected by fasting and "natural living," her way of saying natural eating and sensible living.

At our suggestion, a young couple longing to have children yet still childless after years of marriage, had tests to reveal their body levels of vitamins, minerals and amino acids. They were both woefully lacking in many nutrients. A few months after they abandoned their largely prepared and processed foods, drank distilled water and adopted an exercise program which included swimming and walking, the young woman conceived and later gave birth to a well formed, robust baby boy. They now have three of the healthiest small children we know of. They have passed the word along to others, they say, who have also benefited.

Mainly overlooked is the fact that the father contributes half toward the child—his weak characteristics as well as his good ones. What if the father uses alcohol, tobacco and drugs and passes these on to the child? If the mother is healthy, the child has a fair chance. But if the mother indulges in some or all of these, the baby has a very poor start in life.

In cattle husbandry, great attention is given to the bull, not just his lineage, but his feed, water and care, as well as that centered on the cow. The best possible calf is planned for and usually produced as a result. Why do people do so much less for themselves?

The nutrients that play a central part in testicular health, sperm viability and production are zinc, vitamin A and the antioxidants, vitamins C and E along with selenium. Deficiency in especially zinc decreases sex drive as well as lowers the sperm count. In experiments it has been found that samples with the lowest prostate zinc had the lowest sperm count. The low zinc group also had the highest number of abnormal and immature sperm. Zinc energizes sperm. Semen zinc levels reliably indicate fertility potential.

We cannot overstress the role of a natural diet, free of coffee, tea, alcohol, decaffeinate, soft drinks, artificial sweeteners, sugar, white flour, too much meat and all other processed foods. Health of parents and that of the baby they plan cannot come from trash and junk. Parents have the choice of whether to produce a healthy family, a weak one, or no family at all.

INSECT STINGS, BITES AND POISONS: Many people needlessly die from bee sting and from other insect bites. It has been noted that people with nutritional deficiencies are more susceptible to these poisons. They are also the ones the insects, particularly mosquitoes, choose to bite.

The late Dr. Fred R. Klenner of Reidsville, North Carolina, pioneered the administration of large doses of vitamin C, both orally and intravenously for all kinds of poisonous creature bites and stings. Patients recovered in hours, in contrast to patients treated with orthodox drugs for black widow spider, bee and hornet, rattlesnake and highland moccasin. They suffered long and painful recoveries. He also reported persons taking high doses of vitamin C were much less affected by the poison of bites.

We heard a lecture about insects, such as mosquitoes, preferring to bite persons deficient in zinc, magnesium and B6. We paid little attention until finally regaining robust health after the many years of illness. One day after we'd settled in our condominium in Mexico, we noticed mosquitoes weren't biting Elizabeth. We and our physician knew that her body had overcome B vitamin and mineral deficiencies, especially zinc, but mosquitoes avoiding Elizabeth proved it to us. However, mosquitoes still like to bite people sweating from extra exertion, zinc or no zinc.

Biological scientists have long known that predatory insects pester the weaker, less healthy animals. How could we have thought such a condition did not apply to humans?

For relief of a sting or bite, rub with vitamin C crystals or crushed tablet or salt; or fresh cut onion or garlic; or freshly made wheat grass juice; or fresh aloe vera or comfrey juice. (See also BEE STINGS.)

INSOMNIA inability to fall asleep.

Insomnia has plagued peoples of the world for countless centuries. A king of old offered half of his kingdom to anyone who could cure his insomnia without doing harm to his body. He muddled through a long life of poor sleep patterns, never finding anyone to take his standing offer.

Insomnia continues to afflict untold numbers. Despite the many modalities and methods of treatment, mankind has still not solved the riddle. However, when the cause is discovered and can be eliminated, insomnia is usually no more.

Here are some common causes: eating too much; eating refined sugar, especially with the evening meal or before bedtime; intestinal gas; flatulence and constipation; indigestion; food allergies; hypoglycemia triggered by food sensitivities (see HYPOGLYCEMIA); food deficiencies such as calcium, magnesium, vitamin D; high blood pressure; a lack of almost any one or part of the B vitamins, especially B6; faulty absorption of minerals and other nutrients; deficiency of the amino acids tryptophan and tyrosine.

An all-natural diet, a good digestion and retiring after an evening of quiet activity is the basis for good sleeping. Many have found that a tea of camomile, lady's slipper, chaparral, peppermint and especially licorice root, catnip or hops is soothing and helps induce sleep. When Elizabeth added 300 milligrams of chelated magnesium to her daily supplement of calcium-magnesium powder or tablets, she not only ended her problem of constipation, she fell asleep faster, could go back to sleep quickly if she awoke during the night, and needed less time in bed. When fighting insomnia, consider taking extra natural vitamin B6 and magnesium. Think also of thiamine (B1), B3, B12, vitamin C, inositol and L-glutamine. They have all been found to be natural tranquilizers for some people.

Sleeplessness is so widespread that makers of over-the-counter drugs take in millions of dollars from sufferers. Yet we feel that most people, unless gravely ill, can find the cause of their wakefulness and remove it. We have found, too, that with ourselves and with many of our counselees, there is an underlying *physical* cause to the psychological, emotional or mental cause that psychiatrists, psychologists and behaviorists stress as being the sleep stealers. Sit-up, calisthenic, aerobic or mild stretch exercises before bed tend to relax and make you drowsy. Our two-year, in-depth study of insomnia from a mental-psychological approach was wasted as far as improving our ability to sleep. What did help was improving our nutrition and health and doing our exercises immediately before retiring.

INTESTINES, SMALL; PROBLEMS OF: gas, vomiting, duodenal ulcer, malabsorption of nutrients.

Much attention has been focused on the large intestine (see COLON), probably because of the common problems of constipation, polyps, diverticulitis, hemorrhoids, cancer, etc. The function and problems of the small intestine seem to have been neglected. Yet much of the performance of the colon depends on the small intestine. Unhealthy intestines are a blatant invitation to cancer. And it's performance depends on nutrition that includes sufficient magnesium and potassium for good motility.

Symptoms of problems of the small, or upper, intestines range from trapped gas which evidences itself three and one half to four hours after meals, to pain and bloating just under the frontal ribs, duodenal ulcer, pyloric vomiting (vomiting food that has passed from the stomach through the pyloric valve to the upper intestine), and malabsorption of nutrients into the bloodstream.

For many years before Elizabeth was diagnosed as having colon cancer, she had all these symptoms from time to time. However, she had trapped gas as frequently as two or three times a week. Four hours after eating she would feel the first symptom of trapped gas and bloat. If it was after dinner, she knew there would be no sleep for the four or five more hours her system needed to finally work the food on down and expel the gas. No one doctor gave her the answer. Through the years, she learned bits and pieces from several, and from considerable study of the medical literature of alternate therapists.

In oversimplified terms, after mastication foods (starches are mostly digested in the mouth, sugars in the small intestine) go into the stomach where hydrochloric acid breaks proteins down to amino acids. After leaving the highly acid environment and passing through the pyloric valve, food goes immediately in the small intestine, a highly alkaline environment necessary for the pancreatic enzymes to continue their part in digestion so nutrients can be absorbed into the blood and lymphatic systems to be carried to and nurture the cells.

If mastication of food is not sufficient to generate enough of the enzyme ptyalin, which in turn stimulates the production of hydrochloric acid in the stomach, proteins, especially animal proteins, are not properly prepared for the next step in digestion in the small intestine. It often follows that people who have insufficient hydrochloric acid in the stomach have too little alkalinity—potassium bicarbonate and sodium bicarbonate—in the upper part of the small intestine. The fact that they may take hydrochloric acid with each meal to help the stomach do its job doesn't necessarily mean their food will be properly digested further down the line. One deficiency tends to beget another. In this case, not enough of the alkalizing salts in the small intestine. Elizabeth's own nutritionist physician suggested potassium bicarbonate and sodium bicarbonate as possible digestive aids but did not tell her how to take them. It remained for us, some years later, to read the *Appendix for Physicians in Brain Allergy,* by William Phillpott, M.D. He said to mix one part potassium bicarbonate with two parts sodium bicarbonate and take from two-thirds to one teaspoonful, thirty to forty-five minutes after eating. Elizabeth had trained herself to chew foods thoroughly (forty-five to 100 times a bite). She had adjusted her dosage of betaine hydrochloric acid to fit her stomach acid needs for good digestion. She has practically no stomach acid, a condition existing most of her adulthood. Until she discovered the bicarbonate salts, she lived a quarter of her life with mild to moderate, sometimes severe, indigestion.

After months of the treatment and learning *never* to overeat, Elizabeth was able to taper off the bicarbonates and lower the dosage of betaine hydrochloride by one tablet. She praises the Lord for Dr. Phillpott and his simple, natural remedy. It set her on the last lap to good health. It has helped so many people who, like Elizabeth, went from internist to internist without learning the cause or the treatment for their unremarkable gas and indigestion problem.

When the diet, the digestion and the absorption are greatly

improved, diverticulosis, rectal polyps, hemorrhoids and colitis tend to disappear. That's what happened to us. Naturally bulky food (no extra wheat bran), did it for us. It can do it for you. Use the persistance, the patience, the faith God gives to all.

IONIZATION IMBALANCE: lack of normal balance between negative ions and positive ions in the electrical charge of the air.

Ions are electrically charged molecules of gas. Science has long known about this electrical charge called ionization and that it is vital to the creation and health of all life. When negative and positive ion balance is distorted, we humans become physically and mentally ill with from mild tiredness and irritability to digestive disorders, headaches, deep depression, even suicide.

The accepted ratio of ions on a beautiful, healthful summer day is five positive ions to four negative ones. In cities and industrial areas, negative ions are in short supply or absent; while negative ions in right proportion abound near the sea shore, streams and lakes, and in forests.

There are areas in the world where certain seasons of the year send positive, ion-charged currents of air over the land that cause mild discomfort to three-fourths of the populations and real suffering to the remaining fourth of "weather sensitive" people. The Santa Ana winds of Southern California, the Foehns of Switzerland and southern Germany, the Sharav (or Hansin) of the Middle East around Israel, the Chinooks in Western Canada, the Bitter Winds (Indian mythology name) from northern Arizona down into Mexico are all infamous winds, spreading every annoyance from physical and mental malaise to intense suffering. Where the dry Foehn winds blow down from the Alps in fall and early spring, the increase in family fights, car accidents, plane crashes, murders and suicides is called Foehn sickness. Doctors in such regions have learned the incidence of bleeding goes up eighty percent in surgery cases during "bad" wind seasons.

A deleterious excess of positive ions has been created by man in modern environments. Cars, trains, buses, air conditioned buildings, overinsulated and sealed homes, and airplanes are all enclosures with a woeful lack of negative ions. Man literally makes the air sick. Without a sufficient supply of negative ions for balance, people may become lethargic, mentally sluggish, suffer stomach pains and indigestion, headache, depression, double vision, neck pains, poor appetite, temporary impotence and frigidity.

Ion balance is affected by conditions such as moonlight, (above ground vegetables as lettuces, beans, broccoli, actually grow better when planted during full moon because of more positive ions at that time), rain and stormy weather. It is all very interesting to learn about. A fascinating little Bantam book, *The Ion Effect* by Fred Soyka with Alan Edmonds, will give you much information and two or three hours of quality entertainment.

There are ionizers on the market for purifying and balancing the air in your home and car. Health oriented and special equipment shops sell them.

IRRADIATION (of Foods): the application of radiation to foods to destroy insects and bacteria.

The Food and Drug Administration (FDA) of the federal government is favoring the use of irradiation, proposing to substitute it for use of the now-banned pesticide, ethylene dibromide (EDB). But many consumer groups, scientists, nutritionists and biochemists are bringing up some disturbing facts and questioning the safety of irradiated foods. They fear what will happen to the health of consumers over a long period of time.

It has been fairly well established to date that irradiation does not make foods radioactive because of the comparatively low levels of irradiation used. But with irradiation, radiolytic products are produced in foods, products that are foreign to nature. The question is, how will the body handle this foreign matter, chemically distinct from those found in natural foods?

An example of something thought to be harmless when it was introduced, okayed and universally accepted was homogenized milk. But xanthine oxidase (XO), an enzyme in milk, is broken down when homogenized. It is so fine the body cannot excrete it as is possible in the large molecular state of natural milk. Instead it is absorbed into the bloodstream, attacks the heart and collects on the artery walls. Dr. Kurt Esselbacher of Harvard Medical School says that homogenized milk is one of the major causes of heart disease in the United States today. A number of German heart specialists and many other United States physicians agree. When unhomogenized milk is consumed, the body excretes the XO, a harmful substance if left in the body. With the consumption of homogenized milk, the toxin XO *stays* in the body. The harm to millions is staggering.

Are we facing a similar situation in having irradiation forced upon us without conclusive research into its possible harm?

Here's what's being said by the concerned and informed:

Even the FDA, which seems to be advocating it, says: "Ionizing radiation, like other forms of energy used to process foods, causes chemical changes. The chemical reaction does not involve the atomic nuclei of food and, therefore, does not cause any radioactivity, *but the reaction may produce molecules that are chemically distinct from those found normally in food.*"

We are assured the food does not become *measurably* radioactive. But even minute amounts of radioactivity are accumulative.

Research done in the United States, India and Russia show adverse effects of irradiated foods on animals, namely abnormal white blood cells; irradiation produces more aflatoxin poison than there is in nonirradiated foods. The Environmental Protection Agency rates aflatoxin 1,000 times more carcenogenic than the EDB now banned! The offspring of insects fed irradiated chicken bits had increased death rates.

Here are some one liners from research findings on irradiation of foods: such foods affect the metabolic reactions in organisms; growth rates seem to be affected; hydrocarbons are formed; individual amino acids (proteins) are disintegrated, each into a different substance that is *not* an amino acid, and is foreign to the body. Additionally, the quality of fat suffers enormously with toxic substances being developed; lipids (meats), very sensitive to irradiation, produce breakdown products that have repulsive odors; carbohydrates can be disintegrated into highly toxic compounds producing substances injuring cell division and probably hereditary structures; enzymes, especially in meats, often develop high activity which calls for special treatment; vitamins are destroyed. Industry hopes to add them after irradiation. Unfortunately, their biopotency is altered.

Are we facing a situation similar to the one when phosphate and aluminum industries had quantities of waste to dispose of and, through massive propaganda, foisted toxic fluoride on an uninformed public? Selling the food industry nuclear waste would take care of the government's and industry's enormous problem—and at a fat profit.

JAWS, UNDERDEVELOPMENT OF: nutritionally starved.

When too many sweets are ingested, facial bones of children are underdeveloped and the jaws remain so small that teeth crowd together. A narrow jaw bone is not inherited. It results from malnutrition of the mother during the first six or seven weeks of pregnancy. Very little development takes place during the rest of the prenatal period and in early childhood. Excessive sugar inhibits this growth and development. What runs in families is not narrow jaws, but customs of eating nutrition-deficient foods. Sugar also prevents the absorption of calcium, leaving the jaw too weak for optimal health. Why is jaw development so important? The jaw is the strongest joint of the body. The stronger the jaw, the more it can masticate course, fibrous foods. And the more it is used, powerfully, the more the brain is stimulated and kept active. Good nutritious food, from the time of conception, makes good, strong jaws. And strong jaws help to make strong, intelligent, healthy people.

JOINT PROBLEMS: arthritis and gout.

Arthritis and gout cause a great percent of pain in joints. When not well assimilated or ingested in excess, calcium is laid down as small crystals in the soft tissues around joints causing pain during movement. This is known as arthritis. Gout is similar except the crystals in the soft tissue are uric acid that has failed to be converted into urea and ammonia and excreted by the kidneys. Both kinds of crystals weaken the joints and cause pain because the crystals are literally like needles and jab nerves with movement.

Many people first have joint problems in the knees. It is not only the largest joint, it bears the weight of the entire body. It's bending movement is controlled by some of the strongest of our muscles. Therefore, if any crystals at all are present, pain and/or weakness is almost immediate.

"Bad knees" among many young athletes has been on the increase. The answer is usually in the diet. For good bones, children and teenagers are all too often encouraged to drink lots of milk. Not only is it homogenized (the cream molecule distorted and broken up, making it foreign to the body and becoming a harmful toxin rather than a nutrient), it provides too much calcium for the amount of magnesium and panto-thenic acid obtained.

Our friends' eighteen-year-old son had such painful, swollen knees the doctor wanted to operate on them. The doctor advised surgery to "see what is causing the problem." They were not willing to permit an operation, feeling something less drastic and more constructive should be the answer. Together we worked out a nutrition program they attempted to adopt for him.

Since he downed a ten-ounce glass of milk with and between meals, consuming as much as two quarts a day, he was set in a habit of drinking liquids. His mother offered him apple juice, tomato juice, freshly made carrot, cabbage, and celery juice, cranberry and pineapple juice. They decided to leave off citrus juices which contribute to an arthritic condition. Here's what they gave him: fresh vegetables, fruits, sprouted seeds, legumes, cereals, soaked nuts, cornbread, buckwheat pancakes, rye bread, amaranth stove top muffins, brown rice, millet, oats and pearl barley for cooked carbohydrates, and dried fruits and honey for his sweet tooth (no table sugar or commercial syrups). He also took two tablespoons of primary yeast (he would only take the pills, ten tablets to equal that amount), ninety milligrams of zinc (he had white spots on his fingernails), 250 milligrams magnesium gluconate or oxide twice daily, 200 milligrams potassium chloride daily, fifty milligrams pantothenic acid with meals and manganese. For a week or two he took twice the amount of manganese suggested on the bottle, then cut back to the dosage recommended on the bottle.

In a matter of days the young man had no knee weakness or pain. Occasionally he would revert to taking his beloved milk then soon have twinges in his knees enough to remind him of what he was doing wrong.

Since this experience, we have passed the word along both to individuals and to lecture audiences. The feedback attests to some good results and grateful people who thank God they were reminded of His way, the natural way, to take care of health problems.

JUNK FOODS: victuals nutritionally depleted by overcooking, processing and/or chemical additions.

Junk foods may taste divine but they are hellish to digest and expel. Most experts agree that along with sugar and white flour products, processed meats such as sausages, salami, weiners, lunch meats, ham, bacon, etc., are the worst of the junk or trash foods. The animals are fed antibiotics and given estrogen.

Before, during and after slaughtering and preparing for market they may be injected with tranquilizers, bleeding agents, color preservers, tenderizers and preservatives, then dipped in formaldehyde solution. The fat of the meat harbors the poisons of the animal during growth. Such ingested fat is impossible to digest well and gives poisonous overloads to the liver, the greatest detoxifier of the body.

The most nutrition-depleted foods are sugar, white rice and all white flour products like bread, rolls, pastries, cookies, cakes, doughnuts, and pastas. White flour has only fifteen percent of the nutrients present in whole grain flour. Sugar has no nutrition. It has only naked, dangerous calories.

Prepared, packaged edibles are trash food because they are robbed of much of their nutrition. Potato chips are a good example. Most pets won't eat them unless they're as under-nourished as their owners. Instant potatoes, packaged macaroni and cheese, etc., are classic examples of nutrition-robbed, additive-saturated foods. They usually contain artificial flavor and/or coloring, preservatives and goodness knows what.

All cola drinks, soda pops and so-called fruit "drinks" are trash, especially when taken with meals. The extra liquid interferes dangerously with digestion and assimilation of food. They have artificial color and/or flavor, they are carbonated (bad for the stomach), and contain sugar and/or artificial sweeteners which are all proven to be deleterious to health, even addictive. As a matter of fact, we are rapidly becoming a nation of cola addicts. Aspartame (NutraSweet), a classic example of junk food, can cause seizures, deep depression, headaches, mental problems, neurological problems, birth defects and visual impairment. Arizona is trying to get a restraining order to prohibit the FDA from continuing to allow Aspartame as a food additive.

Homogenized milk is another junk food. The cream molecule is so fine it cannot be digested and ends up stuck in the arteries. It is a great cause of atherosclerosis.

The majority of teenagers in America today eat a mono-tonous diet of only nineteen foods, most of them cooked and processed, with little or no fresh fruits and vegetables. Primitive man ate fifty to 200 different foods through the course of a year. Today's youngsters are already unhealthy with all sorts of early signs of degenerative disease showing up. Unless they change soon to a more nutritious diet, they have little chance of optimal health.

JUVENILE DELINQUENCY: irresponsible, wayward, even erratic behavior of teenagers.

Studies of juveniles in correction institutions show their sugar intake to be over 400 pounds a year! The average person in the Unites States eats 126 pounds. Adult criminal offenders in one large institution averaged 456 pounds a year.

Such extreme amounts of sugar every day leave little capacity for nourishing foods. Malnutrition is inevitable. Moreover, the massive stimulation of the naked calories plays havoc with the brain and nervous system. Behavior not only can become erratic and dangerous, it all too often does.

Adult correctional institutions have, as an experiment, given adequate natural nutrition to inmates. In all such programs, the behavior of the inmates improved, they were more calm and cooperative and served less time before being paroled. Despite this, decision makers for those institutions discontinued the good nutrition programs as being too "costly." Yet studies have been made of those costs against the extra cost of keeping inmates a longer period of time. The nutrition way costs much less.

Again, we must report that in areas of the world where refined sugar is a scarce item in the diet and processed foods are practically unknown, there is little or no juvenile delinquency. Not only that, birth defects, mental retardation, insanity and senility are practically unknown.

The American public must resist the false voice of much of the processed food advertising if there is to be improvement in health.

KIDNEY PROBLEMS: nephritis (Bright's Disease) which is inflammation/infection of the kidneys; also kidney stones and kidney failure and bladder infection.

Lately some experts believe that kidney disease may be a result of inadequate nutrition, air pollutants and toxic additives in foods. If a fraction of the money spent for research on kidney disease and propaganda for kidney machines was spent on educating the public in prevention through complete nutrition, there would be little kidney problems. Kidney diseases mostly came into being with the advent of processed foods.

An all-nautral diet, mostly raw, with preferably no animal proteins cannot be overemphasized.

In the case of infection, it is best to start with a cleansing juice diet of both fresh fruits and vegetables, especially dark green leafy ones. Cranberry juice is excellent, as are soaked prunes. They help the body to an acid pH which is necessary to stop the proliferation of bacterial infections in the kidneys and bladder. A watermelon diet is also superb; juice the rind and drink it too.

Effective supplementary foods are vitamin C (from five to fifteen grams a day throughout the day); high potassium foods and/or potassium chloride tablets; magnesium rich foods as green vegetables, spirulina plankton, nuts and all kinds of sprouts—seeds, cereal grains, legumes, and yeast with extra B6. Of course cigarettes, alcohol and sugar should be strictly avoided.

The one time Elizabeth had kidney and bladder infections her nutritionist physician guided her to foods that would most quickly give me a pH of 5.0 or 5.5 so that bacteria could not multiply. He advised her to take daily, eight teaspoons of apple cider vinegar in four doses; two glasses (eight ounces each) of cranberry juice, fresh made and sweetened with honey, which is therapeutic for nephritis; (When fresh cranberries aren't available, frozen juice or juice in glass jars will serve well.) a raw diet with lots of greens; and cornsilk and kidney bean pod tea.

Recently a close friend, a huge hulk of a man, called us to say he was suffering terribly from calcium-phosphorus kidney stones. His doctor had advised a second and immediate operation. Our friend hesitated, realizing operations removed only the symptoms, not the cause. What to do! We were able to tell him others had dissolved their stones with an all-natural, mostly all-raw diet plus 500 milligrams of chelated magnesium, ten to twenty milligrams of B6; 15,000 to 20,000 milligrams of vitamin C, and primary food yeast. A week later he called to say he was so much better he had decided against surgery. We were ready to leave for two weeks and encouraged him to carry on.

When we returned he reported having passed "sand and gravel." He had no more pain. Because his employer required him to have a checkup, he had to submit to X-rays. They showed no stones. He is now free of them and a grateful advocate of nutrition for prevention and recovery.

Note: nephritis occurs most commonly among women. Toilet tissue wiping in a forward motion can introduce bacteria from the stool to the canal from where it travels on to the bladder and kidneys.

LETHARGY: see ENERGY PROBLEMS.

LEUKEMIA: an almost uniformly fatal cancerous disease characterized by excessive production of white blood cells usually in greatly increased numbers in the blood, and accompanied by severe anemia and enlargement and hyperactivity of the spleen and lymphatic glands.

A True Story of Recovery From Leukemia as told by her father, Max Gray, Coff's Harbor, Australia:

Sonia Gray was born September 7, 1970, a normal, healthy baby. At the age of four, shortly after having a full spinal X-ray after falling two meters onto the footrest of a children's swing set, her health deteriorated. Two months later she began to bruise readily, was easily upset. For another four months she gradually got worse, losing considerable weight.

Early in 1975, we received a copy of the *Cancer Control Journal*. We were so impressed, we ordered all back issues. In Volume 2, Number 1, was the information we needed. (Little did we then realize how important that Journal was going to be.)

We consulted our local general practitioner who ordered a blood test. The results were devastating: Leukemia. A second test a few days later confirmed the report.

Between the two tests I reread the article, "Megascorbic Therapy for Leukemia." My wife and I agreed to try this natural treatment. Our doctor wanted to send Sonia to a children's hospital in Sydney for orthodox treatment. However, we rejected this method, feeling if we let her go, she would never come home alive. It was a terrible decision to make. It placed full responsibility on us instead of the doctor.

Seeing we were determined, the doctor agreed to monitor Sonia's progress. We started immediately with the natural treatment on our tiny, thin five-year-old, by eliminating all junk food, red meat and anything containing sugar. Her diet consisted of white meat of chicken, fish, raw and steamed, partly cooked vegetables, almonds, sunflower and pumpkin seeds and plenty of fresh fruits. At the same time I started her on megavitamin therapy, increasing initial doses to optimum dosage as quickly as possible. Luckily Sonia had no reactions or allergies. The daily dosages were established at the following: Vitamin C 20,000 milligrams; vitamin B complex, 200 milligrams for the B vitamins except Folic Acid which was 100 micrograms; and B12, 100 micrograms.

Three weeks after beginning the vitamin treatment we had another blood test. It showed a change for the worse. However, we persisted with the diet and supplements for three more weeks, agreeing if Sonia was no better she would go to Sydney for orthodox treatment. At the end of the six weeks period a fourth blood test was done. There was no sign of leukemia. Her blood had returned to normal. It was a miracle!

We continued with the large doses of vitamins for some months before slowly cutting down. We found that Sonia became tired and pale if she didn't get enough vitamin C.

Even now, 1978, Sonia still has her daily dose of supplements which includes a gram of vitamin C for each year of age (eight). There is no sign of leukemia, the dread disease that was triggered by X-ray radiation exposure over her torso and neck when she was four years old.

LIP BLISTERS: see FEVER BLISTERS.

LIVER TROUBLES: fatty degeneration, congestion, sluggishness, liver toxemia, liver enlargement.

The liver is the largest internal organ, with thousands of chemical reactions taking place in it every second of life. It does so many things for the body, space here prohibits listing them. Suffice it to say, it is an all-important organ—detoxifying, recycling, converting, storing, destroying harmful wastes, etc. It pays to nourish the liver well and refrain from poisoning it with alcohol, drugs, tobacco, bacteria, toxins and pollutants. Any of these can cause liver damage, then scar tissue which in turn inhibits liver function. With impaired liver function there can only be impaired digestion assimilation.

Other things can damage the liver: cooked and rancid fats and oils, chemical additives in foods as artificial color, artificial flavor, preservatives, artificial foods as cream toppings, most ice creams, chlorine and fluorides in water, environmental poisons, and synthetic vitamins. Liver damage inevitably follows all poisonings. Strong spices as black pepper, mustard, horseradish, salt and sugar should all be eaten sparingly, or not at all. They too, can damage the liver.

Perhaps no greater thing may be done for the liver than to help it cleanse itself. There are several ways that are painless and effective. A doctor friend of ours says eating grapefruit four times a day—all you want—for a day or two is fantastic for liver cleansing. A Chinese-American doctor we know prefers the grape diet for a week or so. We were delighted with the results of a three week watermelon diet. We juiced the rind and made a milky drink in the blender of the seed and some melon meat and strained, then drank it. Still another nutrition-practicing M.D. friend finds the following very effective: mix juice of ten lemons in two quarts water, sweeten with raw honey and drink a glass every two hours, interspersed with a glass of green vegetable juice. Include beet tops because beets are very good for the liver.

After the cleansing, all fats and oils should be avoided for several weeks, as well as avoiding all canned and processed foods, and strict avoidances of overeating. High quality protein essential for liver repair is found in brewer's yeast (also rich in B vitamins vital for recovery), sprouted grains, legumes and seeds, raw soaked nuts, avocado, raw almond and raw sesame seed butter. Sesame seed is high in calcium, unsaturated oil, methionine and proteins, all especially good for the liver. Raw vegetables and fruits with emphasis on lemon are excellent. Remember that five to fifteen grams of vitamin C is a great liver detoxifier.

We write this from personal experience. We both had serious liver damage, Elizabeth from bad diet and too much radiation from X-rays, Elton from too many chemicals and radiation during years of research in nuclear chemistry/physics. It took years to "pass" the liver test. But we did with God's help. We used Psalms: 103-5. "My youth is renewed like the eagles." It has come about. What a superb blessing!

MALABSORPTION: the lack of ability of the small intestine to digest nutrients sufficiently and get them into the blood stream for transport to all the cells of the body.

Many who have a malabsorption problem don't even know it. One way to find out is to eat beets and watch for red beet juice liquid to come through with the feces. If it does within twelve to thirty-six hours after eating, malabsorption is indicated.

Almost all people with health problems have some troubles with digestion—indigestion, heartburn, gas, malabsorption. For most, an improved diet of natural foods instead of processed ones works wonders. Getting natural bulk into the diet with natural nutrients is all important. Doing so costs less than staying on a conventional diet. But don't take our word for it. Try it and see for yourself. (See also INTESTINE, SMALL.)

MASTICATION: the act of chewing food.

Mastication is not a problem. *Lack* of mastication is the problem. It plagues millions of people. It is even promoted on television commercials. We have yet to see a TV commercial on food consumption that didn't show people biting into the food like ravenous animals and downing it after a few canine chomps. Or shoveling in spoonfuls of soup or pudding with no chewing whatever. Or gulping a whole glass of juice, milk or beer without coming up for air. What an example for our young viewers! Not only is it is bad manners, it's disastrous for the digestion.

Some time ago we made a study of the chewing of twenty-eight people in the relaxed atmosphere of a good restaurant. None observed chewed any bite over twenty-five times. The overall average was eleven. One very obese lady who chewed mashed potatoes *one* time before swallowing and other foods two to six times, caused us to observe other overweight people. They chewed the least and ate the most. It is difficult to overeat when mastication is thorough. If over a period of days you count the forty to sixty "chomps" it takes to masticate each bite thoroughly, you can break the health destroying habit of eating too fast. Nutrition oriented physicians say we should chew each bite at least forty-five times.

It takes great self-discipline to cope with life in our fast-paced country. Maybe discipline is the quality we need to cultivate. Maybe it's enjoyment. Perhaps if we choose the natural foods God planned and provided for us, then in thankfulness take a few extra moments during meals to show our gratitude by prolonging the wonderful taste through mastication, just maybe we could break a bad habit—the pernicious, health-destroying habit of gulping food into our stomachs. It takes more food to satisfy our appetite when not eaten slowly, enjoyably. In other words, when we eat slowly, we eat less. Eating too much is gluttony and gluttony is a sin.

MEMORY LOSS: inability to recall.

There is nothing more frustrating than a gradual, insidious loss of memory. Experiments have been made with seniors in retirement, nursing, and rest homes who were given a highly nutritious, natural diet. There was improvement of the memory of from thirty to seventy percent, depending in part on the severity of the memory loss, the length of time of the "poor" memory, and the health status of the person.

Worry and tension—both negative emotions—also stifle blood circulation to the brain, thus contributing to poor memory and inhibited intellectual activity. Negative thoughts and emotions are closely associated with fear, which causes nervous exhaustion and mental fatigue. They restrict blood circulation to and through the brain. Faith and eagerness are the natural conservators of brain energy and the result, happiness, is the secret of mental and nervous economy. The joyous soul can perform twice the mind and body work with half the expenditure of mental and physical energy. Faith begets energy and brain function. Fear weakens the brain centers.

Faith, proper food and exercise can reverse much of the deterioration of our senior population. The natural diet of unprocessed, at least seventy-five percent raw foods, and these food supplements may help in maintaining and restoring memory: lecithin granules (at least one tablespoon a day); brewer's yeast; spirulina plankton; sesame seeds (budded, blended); and periwinkle tea. Choline, like lecithin, a precursor for acetylcholine, is considered by many therapists to be helpful. Poor memory people have been found to be quite deficient in this nutrient.

Since memory depends on good brain function and that function depends on an adequate supply of good blood, it is well to do everything possible to get that blood to the brain: elevating the foot of the bed two or three inches; exercise; walking; learning to do foot reflexology; a hot sitz bath with epsom salts; alternating hot (one minute), cold (two minutes) foot bath; rebounding on a home trampoline of the rebounder type, a good taut, round one. This is excellent for the circulation, as is the backswing if you don't have high blood pressure.

It is interesting to note that people in areas of the world where processed foods are not eaten, where the diet is natural, mainly raw, do not suffer memory loss. They live to be old with all their faculties intact.

MENSTRUATION: the cyclic discharge of bloody fluid from the uterus.

Menstrual disorders cause all sorts of symptoms—cramps, headache, backache, water retention, breast tenderness, tension, tachycardia, etc. They are common but not normal. Women in small so-called third world countries who live close to nature, eat all-natural foods and get plenty of exercise through hard physical work, suffer little or not at all during their monthly period.

Menstrual problems are often brought about by poor nutrition that leads to hormonal dysfunction and a general run-down condition. There is commonly a deficiency, especially of vitamins E and B6, and magnesium, calcium and zinc—all of which can be gotten from unprocessed foods and/or natural supplements.

An all-natural diet, mostly raw, with enzymes intact, cannot be overemphasized. And natural supplements help many: brewer's yeast for the B vitamins, especially B6, and for complete protein; spirulina plankton, especially for B12, the antianemia factor; kelp for minerals, especially iodine; black strap molasses; sprouted whole grains and nuts.

No smoking. It aggravates menstrual problems. Ideally, no refined sugar or alcohol. Both contribute the lion's share of hypoglycemia reactions.

During World War II, menstrual disorders were cut by sixty percent where employers required of each female employee a simple, two-minute exercise. Before starting work, women were lined against a wall with heels, buttocks, shoulders and head touching that wall. In this position they pulled inward and upward with their stomach muscles as much as possible, while inhaling, then holding the position as they exhaled. That is all. That simple exercise pulled the uterus into position.

A second exercise was given to stubborn cases with an out-of-line uterus. In the bicycle position (hips held in the air with elbows on the floor, hands on hips), the legs were pulled apart at the hips so that air was pulled into the uterus, bringing that organ into line and leaving a good restful feeling. That single exercise ended Elizabeth's cramps. What a blessing was that bit of knowledge!

METAL POISONING: sometimes called toxic disease.

The most common, poisonous metals in the body are lead and mercury, with cadmium, Strontium 90 and aluminum close behind.

Lead is increasingly found in food, water and air. It mostly comes from leaded gasoline but is also present in ceramic glazes, paints, amalgam tooth fillings (silver), and in industrial products. It is cumulative. It can cause strange and severe illnesses and death.

Mercury, universally present in our environment, has contaminated food supplies, soil and water. A deadly, cumulative poison, it can damage the central nervous system, the brain, enzyme activity, kidneys and liver. It can also cause blindness and paralysis.

Nuclear explosions and tests have contaminated the whole globe with Strontium 90. Scientists say all people now have dangerous amounts of radioactive Strontium 90 in their bones where it stays throughout life. Like X-rays, it emits radioactive rays. Sarcoma of the bones, anemia, leukemia and other cancers are linked with Strontium 90 poisoning. Vitamin C in large doses (five to ten grams a day) is known to be an effective detoxifier.

Aluminum poisoning may result from aluminum cooking utensils, deodorants, the use of aluminum wrap directly contacting food, baking powder and over-the-counter antacids. Accelerated aging and Alzheimer's disease (senility) are believed to be caused by aluminum, as is slow learning in the young.

Cadmium, beneficial in trace amounts as it occurs naturally, is another environmental pollutant. It is extremely toxic. Present in many brands of lubricating oil and in gasoline, it is emitted into the air by automobiles. It is in smog. Shellfish and animal livers have concentrated cadmium and are dangerous to eat. Tap water, both from galvanized and plastic pipes, has cadmium from water standing in those pipes, hot water more than cold. (We are advised to cook with and drink only cold water after letting it run awhile.) Cadmium is also in the enamel of pots and pans and is dissolved by the acid in foods. More dangerous than lead, it can cause even more damage to your health—heart disease, high blood pressure, anemia, emphysema, kidney damage, cancer, chronic bronchitis, etc.

Acid rain, another source of metal poisoning—nickel, lead, zinc, cadmium, manganese—pollutes our streams.

What to do?

In all cases, eat an optimal diet of live, organically grown foods and drink distilled or pure well water, bottled if possible. Live in clean air. Choose natural fiber clothing and household furnishings. Vitamin C and calcium are specific detoxifiers. They chelate aluminum out. Brewer's yeast, hydrochloric acid, spirulina plankton and sea plants such as sea lettuce, dulse, and kelp, all help. According to one physician friend, an internationally known allergist, selenium offers the greatest help in tolerating chemical toxicity. Yeast has abundant selenium.

MENTAL PROBLEMS: see AUTISM.

MINERAL DEFICIENCIES: a shortage of mineral or minerals that contributes to subnormal function of a part, parts, or all of the body.

Volumes have been written on the role of minerals in body metabolism. Yet mineral deficiencies causing or contributing to problems from birth defects to degenerative diseases to mental failure are rampant.

Why is this so? Soils are leached of their original supply of minerals. Processing of foods takes out as much as ninety-nine percent of the minerals. Cooking, and destroying the cooking water, leaves the part served woefully lacking in minerals and other nutrients. Drugs often block the body's utilization of certain minerals. Medical science has been painfully slow in updating medical textbooks on the part minerals play in health and resistance to disease. As a result, mild to critical mineral deficiencies may not be recognized or prescribed for. This regrettable situation may be the missing length in the chain of treatment that leads to healing.

It behooves us all to see that we get adequate amounts of every nutrient. Fresh, raw, organically grown foods and sea plants as kelp, sea lettuce and dulse all help when given. Take them in natural balance, which is all important.

MOTION SICKNESS: mild to severe nausea and even vomiting.

Some motions that bring on the sickness are car riding, especially in the back seat; boat riding; flying in inclement weather that causes the plane to rock; swinging; amusement park rides, etc. Health professionals are reluctant to suggest probable causes.

Recently many have picked up on the findings of those who have tried vitamin B6 and magnesium, two nutrients that work together. This inadvertently discovered treatment worked for us, and has since benefitted for many we taught in self-help classes, seminars and workshops. Some people have not been helped by taking tablets of vitamin B6, which at best are ninety-five percent synthetic. Without having sufficient, accompanying micronutrients, the body may not be able to metabolize (utilize) it.

Most of her life Elizabeth suffered motion sickness in the back seat of the car on an extended drive, in a plane during "choppy" weather, or in a boat in rough water. But in all the years of taking primary yeast, bee pollen and spirulina plankton she has never experienced motion sickness. There are drugs that relieve motion sickness but they mask the symptoms rather than deal with the cause.

MOUTH PROBLEMS: sore mouth, outside and in, possibly caused by drugs, allergies to food, or vitamin deficiencies, particularly vitamin C and B complex.

Improving the nutrition by including foods high in these nutrients and taking primary yeast and/or spirulina plankton and extra vitamin C usually allow these conditions to clear up in days or a few weeks.

Fresh pineapple causes many people to have a raw tongue and sore mouth. This is rarely an allergy. Rather, it points up a vitamin B deficiency and an added need for magnesium. When the diet includes sufficient of these nutrients, pineapple will rarely cause sore mouth.

MULTIPLE SCLEROSIS: patches of hardening in the brain and spinal cord.

It is claimed by some experts that multiple sclerosis is often just a magnesium sulfate deficiency. A clinic in Germany has for years been helping people to improve, and even get over, multiple sclerosis by maximum nutrition. Early in our nutrition studies we interviewed a twenty-eight-year-old, pretty, healthy, career-directioned, former patient of our nutrition-practicing physician and friend. She had come to him three years before in a wheelchair. Her speech was affected, she had little use of her hands. The most difficult task she faced in her recovery, she said, was to change from the junk food diet of her peers in high school and college. But from the first few days of following the doctor's program, she began to improve. In three years, it brought about her nearly complete recovery.

What she did: ate organic living (raw) fruits and vegetables, mainly those of the cabbage family, beets and sauerkraut; sprouted legumes; grains, seeds and soaked nuts; oat bran soaked overnight and/or sprouted oats eaten raw as cereal with raw goat's milk or fresh fruit juices; raw butter and raw fertile eggs (puncture the big end of the egg, then drop into boiling water for twenty seconds only. This destroys the toxic enzyme, avidin, just under the shell. Break and serve over sprouted cereal grains warmed to 104 degrees and seasoned with butter); sprouted wheat, rye or buckwheat at least once every day; liquid whey from homemade cottage cheese—the orotic acid in it is especially beneficial for multiple sclerosis; and unfiltered, raw honey (no other sweetener allowed). She consumed no processed foods, salt, refined sugar, coffee, tea, chocolate, spices or refined carbohydrates.

This young woman, so radiantly happy, said with great compassion, "My ambition is to tell the world how terrible are the consequences of a processed food diet. I went through college living on canned soups, crackers, processed cheese and candy bars. It's a sure way to degenerative disease. I daily thank God and my doctor for guiding me to the right diet so that my healing could take place."

MUSCLE SPASMS, STIFFNESS, SORENESS: cramps in muscles, charley horses, twitches, tremors.

The most common muscle spasms occur in the legs, feet and hands. However, they can happen in muscles anywhere in the body, as the heart, our hardest working muscle.

Almost every adult at some time in life, has experienced a cramping, jerking muscle. What prevents or stops them? Most physicians, therapists, and nutritionists agree it's calcium and magnesium. Recently they have found vitamins B6 and pantothenic acid are also involved. Potassium, too, plays a part, and possibly manganese.

With health at low ebb a number of years ago, Elizabeth got some relief by taking three dolomite tablets that provided approximately two grams of calcium and one gram of magnesium a day. When she added brewer's yeast that gave her the B vitamins, she had no more spasms. At the same time she had tic douloureaux, which also stopped and has never returned. Occasionally muscle spasms do recur after stress on a trip or heavy schedule, and neglect in taking yeast.

Once when Elizabeth took calcium gluconate, intestinal gas, a common reaction, forced her to try another form of calcium. Knowing about horsetail (shave-grass) tea for silica, she began taking a strong cup of it a day along with calcium and magnesium ascorbate (vitamin C). That combination seems to serve her well.

Many people have come to us asking what to do about muscle cramps and tics. We tell them of several remedies, all of which have helped with the problem of this or that person. Possibilities are: calcium (chelate, gluconate, lactate, citrate, ascorbate), sesame seeds, dark green leafy vegetables, egg yolks; magnesium oxide, magnesium chloride, chelated magnesium, or unflavored milk of magnesia (one teaspoon three times a day); vitamins B6 and B2, brewers yeast, spirulina plankton, sprouted seeds, cereal grains, legumes, whole grain cereals and breads; silica (powder) or horsetail (shave-grass) tea, chaparral tea; raw honey (no more than one tablespoon daily).

Stiff and sore muscles follow overactivity or strenuous use of muscles not in condition. Shoveling off the first snow, or gardening too much on the first nice day of spring, or too strenuous a workout when starting a physical activity program are examples of suddenly introduced, strenuous activity that can cause painfully stiff and sore muscles. The greatest single word of wisdom may be vitamin C. If two grams are taken at the start, and another two grams an hour later, then another two grams at bedtime, muscle stiffness and soreness may be minimal or none at all.

A home accident put two inches of water in our basement a while back. Three of us worked several hours scooping up and carrying out water, lifting heavy objects, moving and piling furniture, all work none of us were "in condition" to do then. We took vitamin C. Our good neighbor assured us he'd be fine without it. Next day, when he could hardly move around, he readily took the extra vitamin C. We, ten years his senior, were fine.

NEURITIS AND NEURALGIA: inflammation of the nerves.

According to *Stedman's Medical Dictionary*, neuritis and neuralgia are simply nerve pain. Although the two conditions may be slightly different, they respond favorably to the same treatment.

They can be caused by metabolic disturbances and numerous nutritional deficiencies of B vitamins (B1, B2, B6, pantothenic acid, B12), poor phospholipid metabolisms, toxemia, etc. All may be relieved by optimum nutrition that is well assimilated.

Allergies impede relief. If a food gives the patient a problem, it invariably shows up in delayed healing or extra pain in an already intensely painful area. For this reason, the muscle test should be given to determine the offending food, then that food avoided.

When Elizabeth was in college a severe sinus infection left her with such intense neuritis and neuralgic pain of the face, eye, ear and mastoid that a few times she experienced brief intervals of semiconsciousness. Cold triggered these attacks more than anything else. To prevent them she designed all sorts of headgear for sleeping and fur caps with a swatch of fur covering the affected sinus. Finally a doctor friend told her to take two to three teaspoons of apple cider vinegar in water four times a day and the neuritis pain would stop in hours. To her amazement, it did. He later explained that when the body pH (the acid-alkaline balance) is too high (on the alkaline side), it is vulnerable to all sorts of illnesses. The neuritis-neuralgia of Herpes Zoster for the same reason began to abate immediately when she took vinegar and applied it topically.

Note: Doctors have found that all patients suffering from virus or bacterial infections, from cancer and from many kinds of severe inflammation, have a high pH of 7.0 or more. The body should be slightly acid as revealed by running a little urine over a bit of nitrozene paper, at the first voiding of the morning. If the paper is 7.0 or 7.5 (purple) there is a problem. If the paper is 6.5, 6.0 or 5.5, it indicates the body is recovering from the infection and energy is returning. Remember that virus and bacteria cannot multiply in an acid environment.

Neuralagia may be caused by nerve impingement during sleep. For instance, a man we know who had severe nerve pain in his arms and shoulders slept with his head on an arm. On a hunting trip an associate commented that the habit was bad for circulation and his skill in handling a gun. When the man forced himself to sleep with his arms outstretched or relaxed alongside his body, there was no more pain.

The Encyclopedia of Common Disease by the staff of *Prevention* magazine reports many similar cases of "sleep neuritis" caused by pressure on the nerves that were completely cured when the cause was removed.

NIGHT BLINDNESS: inability of the eyes to accommodate to darkness or semidarkness.

The person with night blindness literally can see much less

than is normal, or not at all, depending on the severity of the condition. Such a condition indicates a deficiency in vitamin A, usually accompanied by a lack of vitamin C and B2 (pantothenic acid). Two members of our family who had so much trouble with night vision they had to avoid late driving were absolutely ecstatic when their vision improved so much they could drive after dark with ease and confidence. They took all three vitamins in these approximate amounts: 75,000 units vitamin A; ten grams of vitamin C in one to two gram doses around the clock and one tablespoon of yeast morning and evening. In eye problems, vitamin B2 is indicated. Yeast provides sufficient for most, as do sprouts eaten daily. Others have reported being helped by taking only vitamin A or carrot juice. (See also RETINOSA PIGMENTOSA.)

NIGHTMARES: see DREAMS.

NUMBNESS OF EXTREMITIES: a tingling "going to sleep" of hands, feet or other parts of the body, involving the peripheral nerves.

Numbness is a common symptom of vitamin B6 deficiency. It is a real warning to us that either we're not ingesting enough B6 in our food or our intestines (a weak spot) are not functioning well enough for synthesizing B6 from the carbohydrates we eat. By concentrating on more sprouts and not neglecting our yeast-spirulina mix, we soon eliminate the numbness in our hands we wake up with in the middle of the night, especially if we also get sufficient magnesium and potassium.

OBESITY: see WEIGHT CONTROL.

OSTEOPOROSIS: see BONE PROBLEMS.

OXYGEN PROBLEMS: see EMPHYSEMA.

PAIN: distressing sensation due to bodily injury or disorder.

A malnourished person is more sensitive to any kind of pain than an optimally nourished one. A nurse we know became so disillusioned with the "nutritionless diet," as she termed it, of the large, respected hospital where she worked for years in intensive care, that she went back to school for a degree in nutrition at a now famous university. She noticed that the patients of doctors who prescribed highly nutritious diets, vitamins C, E, and calcium, suffered far less pain and recovered faster. When she passed this observation on to the hospital, she was threatened with dismissal.

Here are a few solutions for pain that we and others have tried and found effective: calcium with magnesium (two-thirds and one-third respectively) and vitamin B6 for arthritis, menstrual cramps, tension headache, surgery. For pregnancy stretch marks, calcium-magnesium and vitamin E (try large amounts of brewer's yeast—it's good for calcium, fair for magnesium, great for B vitamins). Vitamin E (and some calcium-magnesium and potassium) for heart disease pain. Start with a small amount, gradually increasing to what your doctor recommends. Vitamin E for pain of varicose veins, rubbed on and taken by mouth. Vitamin C for back pain from injury, arthritic deposits and strain. Vitamin C is great for pain in general, from burns through the gamut of infections to stress, cuts, bruises, radiation, chemotherapy and mental-caused pain.

Primitive man got in his diet an estimated eight to twelve grams a day of vitamin C and twenty to thirty units of vitamin E. On a conventional diet, man gets forty-five milligrams of vitamin C and as little as one and one half units of vitamin E. Small wonder there is so much disease when such deficiencies occur!

PANCREATITIS: inflammation of the pancreas, that all-important organ that is seldom mentioned short of diabetes and cancer.

The pancreas is the slender organ to the left and a little below the stomach. Pancreatitis, inflammation of the pancreas, may occur during a deficiency of certain amino acids, vitamin B6 and/or protein. Drugs and chemicals, cortisone and ACTH also can cause the disease, especially when the nutrition has been insufficient. Pancreatitis keeps the pancreas from performing its all-important role of producing certain digestive enzymes and insulin which provide for sugar (glucose) to enter the cells, then be converted to energy. If not needed at once, it is converted to glycogen (body starch) or fat, and stored. To be used, stored fat must have insulin which the pancreas must synthesize.

When the pancreas produces insufficient insulin, the body becomes diabetic. When it produces too much, the body's blood sugar is burned too quickly and the result is low-blood sugar, or hypoglycemia.

If the diet is inadequate—especially in B vitamins (emphasis on B6) and pantothenic acid, vitamin E and vitamin C and magnesium—function of the pancreas and general health go down. Imbalance in sodium/potassium levels contribute. Among the first signs of pancreatic problems may be dark blotches on the face and hands, spreading to the neck and arms if not corrected. (Liver dysfunction can also cause such disfigurement.) When they appear, all attention should turn to natural, mostly raw foods, little salt (sodium), no processed foods, plenty of the B vitamins and vitamin C. Caffeine should be avoided completely. There is a direct link between caffeine and pancreatic cancer.

PARKINSON'S DISEASE: palsy or paralysis agitans; "A neurological disorder caused by postinflammatory or degeneration of the basla ganglia," according to *Stedman's Medical Dictionary*.

This deficiency disease, treated early on, responds well to a completely raw diet, low in protein and high in the B vitamins and minerals, especially magnesium.

We have known several people who suffered this affliction but only one who was willing to change even a little bit. Mainly she quit eating processed foods and took the magnesium we suggested for constipation. This helped so noticeably she got a new lease on life at seventy. Although her hands still trembled slightly, her head has ceased to shake. She had learned to sprout grains, seeds and legumes which became a large part of her diet, giving her a good supply of B vitamins. Because she eliminated the allergy-causing foods we discovered through muscle testing her, she had good energy and took a part time job.

Again, we come back to nutrition for helping the body heal itself. It was made to self-heal. It was all in God's planning.

PIGMENTATIONS PROBLEMS: see VITILIGO.

PNEUMONIA: a viral infection of the lungs or bronchia.

This dread disease, the number three killer in the elderly and number six overall, occurs in all ages. Pneumonia follows a rundown, toxic, low immune condition of the body. Patients tested are found to be almost totally lacking in vitamins A and C, among other nutrients.

An increasing number of physicians are giving intravenous sodium ascorbate (vitamin C) with calcium which increases the value of vitamin C, with excellent, rapid results. Some physicians at Johns Hopkins Hospital have been using vitamin C in this manner for years. Why this spectacular treatment receives only a pinpoint of publicity when its nearly unfailing cure is so miraculous, we do not know. And why the taking of megadoses of vitamin C to prevent flu, colds, and pneumonia is talked down, remains another mystery.

Usually the pneumonia patient is hospitalized for intensive care, antibiotics, removal of water on the lungs, monitoring, oxygen, and so on. Recovery is discouragingly slow unless an optimal nutrition program is immediately adopted.

Having had pneumonia five times, each time subjected to a different treatment, Elizabeth has studied the disease from the various points of medical view and made some interesting observations.

The first time she had pneumonia she was a young woman attending graduate school with Elton and working as a librarian. The critical phase—no wonder drugs—lasted a week; hospital confinement three weeks. Her woman physician saw that she was served mainly fresh fruits and vegetables. (The doctor was humored in her instruction by the male university physicians because she was "a sweet little person.")

The second time Elizabeth had pneumonia, when our children were just school-age, the doctor gave her the "wonder drug" Chloromycetin, which quickly ended the awful lung congestion—but started her long, agonizing health deterioration. It included mononucleosis, constant temperature, digestive problems, arthritis and most of the other things we're writing about in this book.

The third and fourth times Elizabeth had such severe lung infection nobody at the hospital thought she would live. Both of these times God sustained her until she got to her allergy-physician and Christian brother on the Oregon Coast where he gave her the foods she should have, intravenous vitamin C with calcium, and supplements of vitamin A, E, and bioflavonoids. Hospital doctors would not allow her doctor to give her 150 grams continuous drip of vitamin C, the amount Dr. William Phillpott recommends for a person of Elizabeth's size (107 pounds). Since they allowed her doctor to give her only eighty grams, he brought the vitamin in powder form and asked her to take seventy grams around the clock. God helped her during that near fatal first week and ensuing five weeks and brought her out of the dark tunnel where at first she could see no light at all. He had more things for us to learn to do.

The last time Elizabeth had bronchial pneumonia was eighteen months before this writing. A thorough chilling from a sudden cold wind and fatigue when we were hiking, was too much for her low immune system. We were in our condominium and a physician there advised us to fly to our doctor for vitamin C by i.v.

God pressed instructions on Elizabeth's mind. She was to stay and water fast as she had learned to do (see FASTING). And fast she did, nine weary, suffering days. The awful phlegm she constantly coughed up was less after each night's sleep of only four hours. The morning of the ninth day Elizabeth awoke feeling good. The fever was gone. She coughed up only a bit during the day, and considered taking two or three ounces of fruit juice. The temperature was normal. But after reading scriptures on healing and praying she knew God's will. She was to fast until there was no mucous coughed up for a day.

The evening of the tenth day Elizabeth took fruit juice, one tablespoon. How marvelous was that occasion. We held hands and gave grateful thanks to our Lord. Elizabeth was on her way.

Elizabeth has never recovered from any severe illness so fast. It was a miracle of a cleansed, disease-free body restoring its strength with easily digested living foods. In two days she was on her regular eating program of all-raw foods. In three days she walked along the beach. In four she started her exercises and in a week, having gained four pounds, she felt her vigorous, enthusiastic self, ready to meet our son, wife and two children on spring break holiday. They never knew she was just one week past a severe bout of pneumonia.

As with all disease, the real answer is prevention. For preventing pneumonia, think dark green leafy vegetables, yellow-orange fruits and vegetables for vitamin A. (It's not difficult to get 73,000 to 100,000 IU. from a day's living foods.) Think whole grains and sprouted seeds and nuts for vitamin E, necessary for assimilation of A; vitamin C so necessary for countless body functions, especially the immune system; raw fruits and vegetables for minerals; sprouts of grains, seeds and legumes for B vitamins, and other nutrients. It's God's way to keep health and to heal the body.

POISON IVY, POISON OAK: members of a family of toxic plants growing over most of the United States.

It has been found that susceptibility to poisons of plants, insects and animals, seems to be more pronounced in persons with a zinc deficiency. In our family of four this certainly applied. Two of us were very sensitive to poison oak-ivy and later learned we had a zinc deficiency. We also learned, years later, the better the levels of vitamin C in the body, the less the reaction. The body *does* store some vitamin C, especially in the eyes, the adrenals, the pancreas and liver when there is enough ingested and to spare for storage. Sufficient vitamin E and A in the diet also help to protect against poisons.

When number one son gets an itchy rash from poison oak he gets immediate relief from an ointment he makes of equal parts of vitamin E, golden seal and honey. He takes at least twelve grams a day of vitamin C.

When Elizabeth inadvertently contacts poison oak, she treats with bandages soaked with apple cider vinegar alternated with vitamin E from a capsule, and takes twenty grams of vitamin C. All is healed in a couple of days.

POST NASAL DRIP: a mucous discharge from the sinus into the throat.

Experts agree the single most common cause of post nasal drip is allergy, with food sensitivities leading even over pollens and other environmental pollutants.

For many years Elizabeth lived with this nagging problem. She is grateful for guidance in studying and learning Kinesiology. She gives thanks for such pioneers in the field as Dr. Goodheart who "discovered" and put to use this science of the body and to Dr. Diamond and others who continue to contribute so much to that development, then communicate it to the world. Through Kinesiology or muscle testing, she keeps abreast of her allergies and sensitivities when other types of testing, except fasting, pinpoint only a few. By keeping them eliminated, her body is greatly aided in the restoration of near total health that she now enjoys. We have introduced Kinesiology Testing to literally thousands. It is widely accepted and utilized by professionals.

We suggest you study Kinesiology as it is presented in *Your Body Doesn't Lie,* by John Diamond, M.D. (See Bibliography and the section on Kinesiology Testing in the Appendix.) As a pediatrician friend of our says, "Muscle testing is amazingly unerring." Remove your allergens and you probably will remove your post nasal drip if, at the same time, your diet gives optimal nourishment. You've a triumph in store.

PROSTATE PROBLEMS OR CHRONIC PROSTATITIS: inflammation of the prostate gland.

Prostatitis is commonly brought on by a lack of sufficient nourishment in the diet. Zinc deficiency is indicated, as well as deficiencies of vitamins C, B, and A. Experts in nutrition have found turnip seed, ground and eaten, or put in capsules and taken, or made in a strong, "boiled a minute" tea, effective as a treatment.

Two older members of our family suffered prostatitis. One did not change his eating habits and continued with a worsening problem that ended in surgery and death. The other did alter his habits and was completely healed. Although slightly older, he is enjoying health and an active life.

Every day he eats one fourth cup of either raw pumpkin seeds, (the highest vegetable source of zinc) sesame, sunflower, flax seeds or almonds, all rich in zinc. They are also rich in high quality unsaturated fats and proteins, all essentials for a healthy prostate. In addition he eats fresh, organically grown vegetables and fruits, sprouted cereal grains and brewer's yeast. He rarely takes coffee, tea and alcohol, considered to be contributors to prostate disorder, or processed foods. At his physical checkup for an insurance policy a year after his new eat-to-live program, the doctor told him he was among the five percent of men over sixty who have a completely healthy prostate. He is now seventy-five and credits his Lord for guidance and help in bringing about a change of diet.

PSORIASIS: a chronic skin disease characterized by red patches covered with white scales.

Because psoriasis is a metabolic disorder, it responds to a cleansing diet, as a juice fast, or a watermelon or grape diet for two or three weeks.

A thirty-year-old man we know had suffered with psoriasis that covered fifteen percent of his body for fourteen years. He read all the literature we had on the disease and selected his program. Neither grapes nor watermelon were in season so he chose to cleanse with grapefruit each day for two (instead of the suggested one) days. He could not quite bring himself to eat the recommended all-raw, animal protein free diet. But he did give up all dairy products and ate lots of sprouted seeds (sesame, flax, sunflower and pumpkin), raw fruits, whole grains, chemical free Wasa Bread (rye), plain rice cakes, avocado, steamed vegetables and cold pressed vegetable oil. Then he added four tablespoons lecithin granules (later two) a day and 100,000 units of vitamin A which he reduced to 75,000 then to 25,000 as the psoriasis began to improve. Since he lived only a few hours drive to the Pacific Ocean, he hauled glass jugs of sea water for sprinkling his skin daily. Although we were prepared for his recovery, we were amazed at the rapidity in which it came about. In one month the red splotches quit scaling and in two months they were gone.

We must remember to say we tested him Kinesiologically for food allergies. The nightshade family (potatoes, tomatoes, bell pepper, eggplant), oranges, onions, corn, and cooked wheat flour products all gave him weak muscles. He was astonished at these results, and even more so at his immediate energy on leaving them off. He was so impressed by this experience that he quit his job as a chemist in a large plant, went back to school, and became a biochemist so he "can help others with equally distressing afflictions," he says.

Do's for psoriasis:
Eat raw seeds and nuts every day, especially sesame, flaxseeds, pumpkin and sunflower seeds; plenty of raw vegetables; raw fruits, cranberry and apple juice; and take two tablespoons a day of crude, cold pressed olive oil. Apply sea water daily over affected parts; exercise out of doors each day.

Don'ts for psoriasis:
Eat any animal fats (saturated fats), pork, milk, butter, eggs, cheese; processed foods; foods containing hydrogenated fats or white sugar. Don't use soap; bathe more than twice a week; smoke; or use alcohol.

PYORRHEA: periodontal disease, a purulent swelling and inflammation of the gums usually leading to loosening of the teeth.

Pyorrhea is a deficiency disease. It results after calcium loss. Calcium can be lost in the urine, in sweat, in calcium deposits. Chewing is extremely important for bone integrity of the mouth.

Pyorrhea is among the first signs of scurvy, an historic vitamin C deficiency disease. It responds favorably and quickly when the diet is improved to include natural foods and exclude white sugar, white flour and all things made from them. The in-laws of a member of our greater family both had tooth-loosening periodontal disease and made countless, costly trips to the dentist. He recommended, along with several medications, 500 milligrams of vitamin C twice a day. This was fine as far as it went, but they still have some periodontal problem. They enjoy their daily cocktail in the evening, (alcohol, bad for lots of reasons, destroys vitamin C), coffee, sugar sweetened pastries, cakes, etc. And how they worry about their pyorrhea!

On the other hand, two members of our family who had early symptoms of periodontal disease immediately followed a nutritionist/dentist's advice by adopting a natural diet of lots of vegetables and raw fruits and some sprouts, yeast, seeds and nuts. Although these two were considerably older than the first mentioned couple, their gums healed completely. One of the two took extra, organic source calcium-magnesium. Later X-rays showed healthy dense bones.

A by-product of their effort was improved general health and energy for one, and needed weight loss for the other. They continue to take five to six grams of vitamin C, bioflavonoids (called the C complex), spirulina plankton especially for B12 and vitamin A.

Our own gums, once inflamed, swollen and bloody, are those of healthy teenagers, says our dentist.

RADIATION DAMAGE: harm from X-rays, radiation treat-ment, fluoroscopes, scans, etc.

Radiation kills cells and destroys vitamins A, E, C, several of the B vitamins, especially B6, and pantothenic acid, all essential nutrients. At the same time, many damaging substances are formed from malignant and other tissues; the liver must detoxify all these but cannot do so unless large quantities of vitamins C, E, and high quality protein with plenty of methio-nine are provided.

There are hundreds of case examples in clinical records of nutrition practicing physicians giving patients the above vita-mins and nutrients before and after surgery. Records show that these nutrients prevent headaches, vomiting, severe anemia, diarrhea, hair loss and hemorrhaging after the use of radioactive cobalt, X-rays or other mitotic poisons. One east coast hospital gives cancer patients three tablespoons of yeast daily for a week before radiation treatment. They remain free of symptoms. Those not so treated suffered severe nausea and anemia.

Patients given vitamins C, E, and A, plus yeast days before and immediately after chemotherapy and/or radiation do not suffer the usual severe nausea nor do they lose their hair. One young man of twenty-one who had gone through radiation and chemotherapy at seventeen for throat cancer was faced with another pending round of the same and was threatening suicide rather than repeat the horrendous ordeal. Our cousin, his mother's best friend, called and asked what we would do if the young man were our son. We suggested: a five-day cleansing diet of raw fruits; primary brewer's yeast, starting with one teaspoon with each meal and increasing over three or four days to a rounded tablespoon; a teaspoon of spirulina plankton three times a day; 100,000 units of vitamin A, 800 units of E, twelve grams of C. He followed these suggestions and went through the "killing" ordeal with little distress and no loss of hair.

Scars left from injury, burns and surgery are reduced to little or no adhesions after vitamin E has been rubbed on daily. Years ago, a cholecystectomy, appendectomy, abdominal exploratory (a three-in-one operation), none of which Elizabeth needed, left her with great masses of scar tissue. The distress of the itching, burning, painful pulling of the scar at that time was stopped by radiation treatment. Vitamin E internally and topically will do the same while adding to general health—instead of contributing to the destruction of health. The visible scar was long, wide, red and ugly. It still pulled when Elizabeth stood very straight. Soon after the operation she started studying nutrition and learned about vitamin E. The results were amazing. In two months the scar greatly shrank and straightened, the purplish red disappeared and lesions no longer pulled when she stood straight.

Radiation burns on a close friend of ours did not heal until she took 800 units of vitamin E, applied it topically, and took extra vitamin C.

Before our number one son had X-rays for an old nose fracture, in preparation for plastic surgery, each day for two weeks we gave him 800 units of vitamin E, 6,000 milligrams of vitamin C, three heaping tablespoons of brewer's yeast, 25,000 units of vitamin A and six kelp tablets. The usual plastic surgery patient, undergoing a nose operation, had to wear the facial bandages from two to three weeks, the surgeon told us. He was amazed that our son's nose was so healed he was able to take the bandages off the fifth day!

Here is one of our greatest gems of information we like to pass on to others: Vitamin E gives wonderful results, not only for burn, radiation, accident and surgery scars—but also for those left by disfiguring acne. As it restores scar tissue, it restores people's self-image, confidence and faith.

There is considerable documentation on many natural foods, supplements and herbs which offer some protection from radiation from such sources as the Russian Chernobyl explosion or leaks from other nearer-to-home nuclear plants. Russian researchers reported brewer's yeast mixed with vitamin C was the most beneficial in offsetting the effects of radiation damage as manifested in nervous and digestive disorders, blood damage, hair loss and other side effects. In Poland children were given iodine which can reduce by eighty percent the radioactive iodine that would go to the thyroid gland. Other food substances that protect from radiation and reduce its damage to the body are Siberian ginseng (no dose established), vitamins A, B6, C, E, folic acid, bioflavonoids, selenium, the amino acids, cysteine and methionine, and the trace minerals copper, zinc, manganese and iron.

Another toxic substance emitted along with a nuclear explosion is strontium 90. It attacks the bones causing Hodgkins disease, bone cancer, leukemia and anemia. The strontium 90 absorbed by the bones can be reduced from fifty to eighty percent by the sodium alginate found in agar-agar, a sea plant food. Take one gram four times a day. The pectin found just under the skins of apples and in sunflower seeds also binds with strontium and takes it out of the system.

There are no known drugs to protect against or rid the body of radiation. But there is good nutrition. We can all see to it we get all the nutrients necessary for maximum health to resist it. And we can make note and keep a good supply on hand of the extra supplements we can take in case of radiation damage from whatever source—X-rays, radiation treatment, fluoroscopes, fallout from nuclear explosion or leak, and so on.

RAYNAUD'S SYNDROME (PHENOMENON): the term applied to the condition of the extremities, usually the hands, when blood leaves. They become a dead white and look like they have been embalmed.

Usually triggered by cold, it must be treated immediately by massage, and when possible, immersing in warm, *not hot* water. Wearing electric mittens in winter will also give some relief.

Little is written on Raynaud's Syndrome, probably because little is known. However, Elizabeth had this distressing problem for several years. It suddenly ended when she corrected her hypoglycemia through discovering her allergies, mainly white table sugar. From the day she quit eating sugar, she had no more Raynaud's Syndrome. Elizabeth was so humbly grateful for this "discovery" that she sent the information, documented by her nutritionist doctor, to the Harvard Medical School. The school had chosen thirty-some students with Raynaud's Syndrome for study and observation in an effort to learn what causes the strange phenomenon. They never answered. Later inquiries into any results they found or conclusions they arrived at failed to get a response.

RESPIRATORY DISEASES: see ASTHMA, BRONCHITIS, EMPHYSEMA, SMOKING.

RESPIRATORY INFECTIONS: see COLDS.

RETINOSA PIGMENTOSA: a slow but eventually total degeneration of the retina causing blindness.

It is preceded by night blindness and other vitamin deficiency symptoms. A young student of psychology and friend of ours asked what he could do for this condition that needlessly causes so much blindness in the United States today. He had experienced night blindness since early puberty. We can't imagine what kind of doctor his physician was *not* to have told him that, first of all, a vitamin A deficiency may be a cause of the affliction. Nor can we imagine a student in his junior year at a recognized university not knowing that eating such food as carrots, apricots and cantaloupe, full of the vitamin A precursor, carotene, help to prevent or alleviate night blindness.

Here is the program he chose for each day after talking to us: vitamin A, 100,000 units (water dispersed because people with this disease do not absorb the vitamin well. He chose to be given it by injection, along with lecithin, oil and bile tablets); vitamin C, 6,000 milligrams; vitamin E, 800 IU; vitamin B2, twenty-five grams; primary yeast, fifteen tablets; vitamin B6, ten milligrams; magnesium, 400 grams.

It was late spring when he started the program. When school was out he went home to work and did not see his doctor until just before he returned to school in the fall. When he reported his eyes were better and what he'd been doing, the doctor said, "You're wasting your time and money taking that stuff. Your eyes got better because you were out of school."

With that, the young man went off his program for his last year in school. His vision steadily grew worse. Not for more than a year, we learned later, did he take any supplements again or return to a better diet. His vision steadily worsened. He could no longer see well enough to drive his car and employed a reader to help him in his first job. Then, on his own, he returned to the program. The last we heard his eyes were not getting worse. We can only pray that he continues and that his sight will improve, as it certainly can with optimal nutrition and persistence.

RUPTURE: see HERNIA.

SHINGLES: see HERPES ZOSTER.

SINUS IRRIGATION: see BRONCHITIS.

SJOGREN'S SYNDROME: see DRY MOUTH.

SKIN CANCERS: malignancy of the skin, usually on the face.

Skin cancers are so common they may not be taken seriously. Yet they are a harbinger of ominous clouds over the status of health, or rather, the lack of it. They often appear before an internal cancer develops, and are usually a different kind. However, the degenerative state that leaves the body vulnerable to skin cancer also leaves it vulnerable to other types of cancer.

When the body is mistreated with poisons from the environment, water and foods and with malnutrition, overeating and overexposure to sun, disease seems inevitable. Skin cancers most often appear early in the degenerative process. They are a powerful warning for us to change our ways. Even though we clean up our diet, environment, and habits, skin cancers tend to stay. Elizabeth's finally healed three to four months after she recovered from colon cancer. Of the three small cancers on her face two disappeared within three and a half months. A fourth one seven years old and as large as a dime on the back of her hand took four months. Over the years several doctors had seen it, each urging her to have it surgically removed. The last one, only months before her colon cancer victory, scolded her soundly. "Get to the best skin cancer specialist you can find and have that thing out. It's damaging the tendons." She expressed thanks and went home. She thought. Cancer around the tendon? Surgery to try to cut it all out? What would that mutilation do to her hand? Leave masses of scar tissue that would cripple it for the rest of her days? She took her chances.

Imagine her joy in God's triumph of healing when the day came that she took the wide adhesive bandage off the back of her hand and the dime-size, flaky cancer scab sloughed off, leaving clean, smooth skin. Only a trace of scar lesions was visible, just enough to remind her frequently to count her blessings.

An elderly gentleman came up to us after we had lectured at The Cancer Control Society, and said, "Elton and Elizabeth, shall I tell you what cured my skin cancers?" We quickly answered yes. "Dry vitamin C fine crystals rubbed on them two or three times a day." How I love that dear man for this precious information. It works. Here's an extra tip: in the morning before applying vitamin C, rub the skin cancers with a bit of vitamin E from a punctured capsule. The C crystals stick better and the E helps in the healing.

Another more recent remedy that worked for Elizabeth is dandelion juice. After a small wart of many years disappeared in ten days by applying the milky root juice of a well-watered dandelion, she began to apply dandelion root juice to skin cancers that had persisted after her last bout of pneumonia a year before. In nine days, the tiny scabby skin cancers were gone. What a miracle! No pain, no inconvenience, no cost. Just His healing through natural means which He gives us free.

SMALL INTESTINE: see INTESTINE, SMALL; PROBLEMS OF.

SMOKING, SNUFF AND TOBACCO CHEWING: addictive, destructive habits harmful to the person doing it and the persons around them.

We all have read the frightening statistics on the curtailed health and life of smokers and tobacco users. We wish only to put forth a few facts that might help the precious victims—the users—and the persons living and working with them.

In our experience there is a sure way to help the addicted tobacco user, coffee drinker, drug user and cola addict to lose his craving for these poisons. That is drinking freshly made juice. It is the easiest way we know of because it is pleasant, the juice is easily digested, it can be drunk often, preparing it occupies the patient, and it is nourishing and satisfying. Most of all, it cleanses the body of all accumulated toxins, the only way to rid the victim of craving. The blood will be purified, the tissues cleaned, the poisons excreted, and *the craving will be no more!* All in two to three weeks.

After this, a diet of all-natural organic foods, whole and chemical free is wise.

One woman told us, "If I'd have known how it was possible for me to give up my two packs a day when I was thirty, I would look my age of fifty years instead of the wrinkled, unhealthy, seventy-year-old I appear to be."

Smoking ages a woman twice as fast, both internally and externally. If a juice diet cannot be arranged, vitamin C, ten to twenty grams a day around the clock could be substituted. A single acupuncture needle applied to the upper part of the ear can dramatically reduce withdrawal symptoms too. A young M.D. acupuncturist we know in Mexico has helped several of our acquaintances in the San Carlos resort area to stop smoking almost painlessly.

SORE THROAT: see COLDS.

SPRAINS, STRAINS, TORN LIGAMENTS: injuries resulting from muscles and tendons being accidentally extended or twisted beyond their normal limitations.

All can heal amazingly fast by a new treatment we've discovered. It's vitamin C topically. Try it. It's working so far for every such injury of those who try it that we know about. First, see a physician if there is any thought of fractured bone. If you're *sure* you've just sprained an ankle or pulled a ligament, here's what can be done: For a newly sprained ankle, strained muscle or torn ligament, dissolve fifty grams of vitamin C powder in two gallons of cold or ice water and submerge the just-sprained foot and ankle. The water should cover the sprain. The cold will reduce the inflammation and the pain almost immediately. Keep foot in water for one half to one hour. Repeat twice a day until sprain is healed, usually in a few days.

Elizabeth's foot, painfully sprained stepping down on the cobblestones of our Mexico driveway, was much better after a single treatment and the good night's sleep she was able to get after the pain-relieving treatment. She could walk on it with no pain if she was careful. After twice daily treatments and the third night's sleep it was healed. We couldn't believe it!

Soon after, a friend did the same thing. But we didn't get the "good news" to her until night. She couldn't walk on the swollen, excruciatingly painful ankle and foot. Her husband had gotten her a crutch from the first aid station after the doctor had verified there was no fractured bone. The doctor had given her pain pills which she did not want to take and ordered her to stay off the sprained foot for two to four weeks as she is a heavy woman. After soaking her foot in vitamin C ice water for an hour, the pain was gone, the swelling was down and she could bear her weight on it. She slept well and had little pain. The sprain was healed entirely in just four days. She never once walked with the crutch. She spread the news by CB radio through the RV camps.

A fourteen-year-old girl whose family we were visiting on an east coast lecture tour was hobbling around on a badly pulled ligament from ankle to mid calf. As she was her school team's star la crosse player, she was disconsolate at not being able to play in the final game in six days. Couldn't we do something? When we said we'd try soaking her foot and leg, out came the mop bucket for the solution. This time we used water about 105 degrees because the wound was two weeks old. After the first hour-long soak she was able to walk without limping. She was radiant with hope. Four more days of the treatment only once a day and she could feel no pain whatsoever. The sixth day she played in the final game. They didn't win but they tied. Her doctor, who had said she could not play or do gymnastics for six weeks, was pleased.

A neighbor with a badly sprained shoulder was warned he couldn't work at his carpentering for at least a month. His wife applied towels saturated with the cold vitamin C water every two or three minutes for at least half an hour. Perhaps her unfinished new cabinets and cupboards and torn up kitchen inspired her to sometimes extend the treatment. At any rate, he was able to go back to finishing the builtins in five days, praising vitamin C all the way.

Note: cold water for new sprains, very warm water for older injuries if inflammation is gone.

SPROUTS: early stage of the water-activated seeds (the bud stage).

When water activates the life force of the seed and it begins to grow (sprout), the nutrition in that seed is doubled many times, sometimes as much as 200. It is amazing to me that so few people have recognized this marvelous energy and health-giving fact and the tremendous economics it brings into play. Besides being a great bargain, sprouts are delicious!

Ponder this startling truth: in sprouts we have our least cost and greatest nutrition. Restated, *we get the most for the least.* Recently a couple in the southwest lived a year on sprouted cereal grains, seeds and legumes and a few fruits in season at a cost of $34.50 a month ($17.25 per person). That was less than one fourth the food cost for the average American at the time. They reported they had good food variety (more than the average person *chooses*), enjoyed high energy, suffered no colds or flu, and passed a physical examination with an "A double plus," to quote the doctor.

Why not give sprouting books for wedding, shower, birthday, and Christmas presents? And buy one for yourself, read it, then try the recipes and *enjoy*!

STRESS, PHYSICAL, MENTAL, EMOTIONAL: body, mind, nerve tension.

In reasonable amounts and at intervals, stress is normal and beneficial to your health. But undue or extra stress from illness, accident, emotional upset, financial problems, work overload, infection, toxins, intense heat or cold, bad posture, faulty metabolism or wrong diet causes fatigue and breakdown of defenses that can speed ageing and start a person on the road to degenerative disease.

Since Eve and Adam were cast out of the Garden of Eden for disobeying God, humankind has suffered all kinds of stress. We lived with fear of wild beasts, starvation, natural disasters, injury, hostile enemies, and death. Smoke from cooking and heating fires in caves, huts, or whatever shelter, was a stressful pollutant, as was severe cold and intense heat. People had to be fit to survive.

There is nothing like a healthy body, good energy and a wholesome attitude to stand up to stress. Nutrition is the main word. An all natural diet of homegrown fruits and vegetables, raw, unprocessed seeds, legumes and cereal grains that sprout, fresh cracked nuts, unhomogenized milk (See IRRADIA-TION), if milk is tolerated, and organically produced animal products if they are eaten. An undernourished body, mind and nervous system cannot cope with stress the way they would if nutrition were optimal. Stress itself does not cause problems. It's the body's failure to cope with stress that causes the problem. That is why Jesus said, "Cast your burdens upon the Lord." Trust in Him to guide you to do what you can, then leave things in His hands.

SUDDEN INFANT DEATH SYNDROME: death of an infant from unknown cause.

Recently experts have found this baffling problem linked to deficiencies of vitamin E and selenium, a trace mineral. These nutrients are very low in both cow's milk and baby formula. Mother's milk supplies much more.

It goes without saying that a prenatal and post natal natural, adequate diet of the mother, and nursing the baby, may well help reduce sudden infant deaths. If nursing is impossible, it should be replaced by one of the commercial brands of milk offering nourishment for the infant that closely resembles mother's milk.

SUNBURN: see BURNS.

SURGERY: that branch of invasive medicine having to do with disease and accidents amenable to operative or manual treatment.

After surgery, nutrition should be optimal. Emphasis should be on easily digested foods high in vegetable protein such as sprouted seeds, legumes, grains, yeast and acidophilus cultured milk.

Dr. Mendelsohn, a pediatrician, lecturer and writer of wide recognition whose interest, among other things, is in warning the public against surgery without at least a second opinion, says ninety percent of surgery performed in the United States is not necessary. Much of surgery seems to be a cop-out. If there is a problem, cut it out; don't bother to find and eliminate the cause. Finding the cause takes time, investigation, study, patience, persistence. Besides, it won't pay for all the costly apparatus surgery entails. The time is coming when very little surgery will be resorted to except in the case of accidents. This trend is evident in the near obsolescence of tonsillectomies (down seventy-five percent), mastectomies (down by half), sinus "windows" and other sinus surgery (down to almost none except for accident cases), and removal of the thymus in small children no longer performed. Knee and back surgery is lessening since the rise of nutrition, Kinesiology Testing, pressure point and manipulation therapies. Heart bypass, made obsolete by noninvasive chelation therapy, is still practiced by the majority of orthodox doctors, even though many of them probably realize its obsolescence. Bypass surgery is big business and big bucks.

Even cancer surgery is off several percent. Patients are choosing alternate therapies, steadily bringing that percentage down further.

At a recent convention of preventive medicine, an oncologist (cancer specialist) admitted to a discussion group of us that heart bypass was obsolete. "Then why are you still doing it?" asked a young M.D. "Oh," the surgeon quickly exclaimed, "My patients want it." What he did not say was that his income would dramatically fall off if he quit performing that drastic operation.

Hardly a day goes by that we don't hear someone's regrets, both wistful and agonizing, for allowing surgery. We have many ourselves. Of Elizabeth's even ordeals, only one was necessary: the Caesarean section when our first son was born. It was a case of placenta previa and was necessary to save his life. The other six were a tonsillectomy, a sinus "window," two D. and C.'s for radical cells, a second Caesarean section, and a cholecystectomy, appendectomy, abdominal exploratory which did immeasurable harm. This triple-header was completely unnecessary. She had only an inflamed gall bladder, a healthy appendix and a poorly performing digestive system from food allergies.

Elizabeth barely escaped two major and two minor surgeries—a hysterectomy, a colon cancer removal and colostomy, a hemorrhoidectomy and the removal of a one half inch in diameter skin cancer on the back of her hand. It was the kind that had tentacles down among the tendons. She was warned that her hand would probably be disfigured and not completely usable because she had let the cancer go too long. Having dedicated her life to her Lord, she trusted Him for the answer. He pressed a "No" indelibly on her mind about those surgeries. Our wonderful Christian physician held faith with her. We daily thank and praise our Lord for guidance in plotting her course to healing the natural way. It is rarely easy but it is joyous because He is always there.

SWEETENERS, ARTIFICIAL: unnatural sweets.

The study of cyclamate, saccharin and aspartame (Nutra-Sweet) continues with no final pronouncements as yet having been made. However, biochemists inform us that the molecules of cyclamate and saccharin are so tiny they pass by barriers that screen out foreign particles not readily digested or eliminated by the body. As with most foreign substances nature did not put in foods, such molecules may act as toxins—poisons. This is bad news for all who seek optimal health.

Aspartame (NutraSweet), hastily approved for use in 1983 by the FDA, is causing all kinds of reactions. The additive is a compound of three components: *phenylalanine* and *aspartic* acid, both amino acids found in proteins, and *methanol* (which is methyl alcohol or wood alcohol), a poison.

Dr. Richard Wurtman, an endocrinologist and brain researcher at Massachusetts Institute of Technology, has found brain changes in people who used Aspartame. Dr. William Pardridge, a brain researcher at UCLA, says behavioral changes could be expected. Indeed, they have come about. Some of the adverse reactions to Aspartame repeatedly reported by doctors and people over the country are severe headache, dizziness, hyperactivity, grand mal type seizures, mental disorientation, speech impairment, fetal abnormalities, loss of equalibrium, menstrual changes, menopause symptoms, irregular heartbeat, chest pains, and elevated blood pressure.

Yet the Federal Department of Agriculture reported in 1985, Americans consumed 400,000 tons of NutraSweet, an average of fifty-eight pounds per person! Each component of Aspartame is associated with a particular form of brain damage when blood levels are raised above normal. This can easily happen to the steady consumer of Aspartame because it is cumulative.

Don't pamper your sweet tooth with potentially harmful artificial sweeteners. Start by skimping the absurd amount of sugar and sweeteners in recipes. Sugar, like nutmeg, is a condiment, not a food. You wouldn't consider putting a cup of nutmeg in a pumpkin pie. By the same token, you shouldn't put a cup of sugar in it either. A teaspoon of each would be far more sensible.

TIC DOULOREAUX: a twitching, involuntary jerking movement of facial, head or neck muscles; facial neuralgia.

Tic Douloreaux is a symptom of any number of problems. It can be a result of lowered health, of degenerative disease, of iatrogenic (doctor/hospital induced) disease, drugs and/or environmental pollutants, pronounced deficiencies or any other condition or factor lowering the health status.

When a neurology specialist advised radiation treatment for a tic under Elizabeth's eye and down into her cheek, she refused. Her sister's best friend, an asthma patient, had so much radiation on a similar tic, her face became horribly distorted. She died a victim of iatrogenic illness, mainly gross overexposure to radiation.

Many years ago, after refusing treatment, the Lord led Elizabeth into an intense and interesting study of nutrition. When she learned the B vitamins with extra B6, vitamin C, the bioflavonoids, magnesium and calcium were involved in nutrition for healthy nerves, she took it as yet another reason for concentrating on an all-natural diet for eliminating her myriad of health problems. The annoying, embarrassing tic disappeared in a matter of days.

Tic Douloreaux is one of countless symptoms and signs of a problem that can be set right when the body is given the repair nutrients it needs to heal itself. Let them be all-natural and undestroyed by fire and heat.

THERMAL BURNS: see BURNS.

THYROID: see GOITER.

TOBACCO ADDICTION: see Smoking.

TONSILLITIS: inflammation of the tonsils, one of the most common afflictions of childhood.

We should not say affliction, for inflammation of the tonsils means that little organ is doing its job as part of the defense team of the lymphoid system, which also includes the adenoids and the appendix. (It's no wonder Elizabeth had colon cancer and skin cancers when one considers her tonsils, adenoids and appendix had all been removed by surgery. In addition, the antibiotic, Chloromycetin had destroyed so much bone marrow she lived with twenty to thirty percent of normal white blood count for years.)

The pediatrician-allergist who fasted Elizabeth in his fasting clinic in Coos Bay, Oregon, treats tonsillectomy patients with vitamin C in megadoses, fresh fruits and/or fresh fruit juices, and bed rest. We found a cloth wet with vitamin C water (ten grams of ascorbic acid dissolved in one pint of cold water) and laid on the throat relieves the soreness, pain, and swelling. After several applications over a period of twenty or thirty minutes, place a semimoist, warm cloth on the throat for fifteen or twenty minutes. Get a second and a *third* opinion if your doctor says the tonsils should come out.

TOOTH PROBLEMS: toothache, oral surgery, night grinding of teeth, etc.

Nothing is more difficult to endure than a toothache. Except for a few caring dentists, many of us would be minus teeth because, in desperation, we would order the tooth extracted to stop the pain.

We wish that some dynamic, universally-accepted person would convince the world's peoples to take care of their teeth through optimal diet, no sugar, cakes, pastries, etc., so they would not have to suffer bad teeth. Prevention of problems begins with parents-to-be so there will be a healthy egg and sperm for a vigorous embryo. But the fact is far from fantasy. Most people have tooth problems that a dentist must care for. The patient may also be having problems from dental stress from a too narrow face, a condition resulting from prenatal B vitamin deficiency.

One of the greatest things we can do for our teeth is eat a mainly vegetarian diet with plenty of complete protein, as in seeds, nuts, legumes, plus such extra rich foods as yeast, spirulina plankton, kelp, sea plants and sprouts. Our teeth stay healthy with the extra chewing of the whole foods. A vegetarian diet is also conducive to a good digestive system free of intestinal putrefaction and bad flora which can cause coated tongue, bad breath, plaque on the teeth and the start of degenerative disease. An all-natural diet person rarely has to worry about cavities, gum disease or bleeding gums, bad breath, body and toilet odors, hypertension, diabetes, arthritis or a host of other problems.

Here are a few things that may relieve pain and distress when you go through ordeals with your dentist.

After oral surgery or extraction of a tooth, take a mouthful of wheat grass juice. It will relieve the pain immediately. Or you can use aloe vera gel (if not allergic to it), or vitamin C water (a solution of four grams to six ounces of water). Do not use ascorbic acid vitamin C. The acid coming in contact with the teeth repeatedly will eventually dissolve the enamel and the teeth will turn brown. Instead use sodium ascorbate

For a toothache before getting to the dentist, use oil of clove on a small cotton swab and apply to the tooth. Or moisten and mash a clove and hold it in your mouth next to the tooth.

For sore gums, natural treatment therapists suggest using oak bark powder put between the teeth, or a piece of hammered oak bark chewed.

If novocaine gives you heart flutters, or makes breathing rapid and difficult, you are probably allergic to it. Have your dentist give you Corbacaine instead. Our dentist discovered the difference the latter makes with Elizabeth and took away most of the dread she had of going to see him. Don't let anyone treat your teeth or your children's teeth with fluoride. Fluoride is a poison and has serious side effects. It is known to cause cancer. And it gives people a false sense of security about their teeth. They continue to eat sugar products believing fluoride will keep cavities from occurring. That just is not true.

Heavy foods like meat, fats, breads, and sugared foods for dinner are difficult to digest and may cause night grinding of teeth, a little recognized but serious problem. If your teeth are wearing down, you should see your dentist. You might need appliances to keep you from further damaging your teeth at night and ruining your bite. A wrong bite can throw your whole system off balance. It can give you headache, vision problems and nervous disorders, to mention a few.

TURISTA: a general, folksy terminology loosely applied to any and all types of diarrhea tourists may get when traveling in any subtropical or tropical country such as Morocco, the Caribbean Islands, the Orient, Northern South America, Central America, Mexico, etc. There are various causes, many of which are overlooked.

1. According to biochemists, there is a difference between the "good" intestinal flora in more northerly climates and the "good" flora of the warm climates. These different flora tend to fight each other, thus causing diarrhea. A return to northern home and foods quickly clears up the problem.

2. "Bad" water is often blamed for the diarrhea "bug." This is not usually the case. Most sizeable towns and all cities chlorinate the water. Most hotels catering to tourists (Mexico is one of the safest countries in the world to travel in) provides pure water— distilled, mineral, filtered or boiled. If not, as may be the case in small, out-of-the-way hotels, management will graciously provide boiled water on request.

3. Americans mostly live in elevations of 1,000 feet to sea level. Their hemoglobin count is thirty percent less than that of people living at 5,000 feet elevation. When Americans go to Mexico City (around 7,000 feet elevation), their hemoglobin count is not sufficient for them to have the energy for activity such as walking a great deal, *and* digesting food. It takes thirty percent of the blood supply to accomplish digestion in the first quarter to half hour after eating. The body has to make a choice. Either it sends much of the blood supply to the stomach, leaving the body so energyless the person has to slow down and rest, or it kicks out the food without it being digested resulting in diarrhea and/or vomiting.

People need to eat lightly, mostly vegetarian fare, possibly with some fish or a bit of chicken, and leave coffee and alcohol alone when at higher elevations.

4. Americans should not eat foods sold by street vendors or small cafes and restaurants that are not regularly inspected by government inspectors.

5. People going from cool-cold climates in summer to semitropical or tropical climates of intense heat to which they are unaccustomed, can become very ill by drinking cold pops and cola drinks in an effort to offset the heat. Such people would save themselves much suffering, and the wonderful tourist land of Mexico great concern and worry if they would drink warm or cool herbal tea and eat only fresh fruits during exposures to intense heat.

A most effective preventive measure for turista is one to three tablets of betaine hydrochloride after each meal. (One for children, two for young adults, and three for middle age to elderly adults.) This is a nutrient (stomach acid) bought at health food stores. Many doctors at long last recommend it. Betaine hydrochloride not only helps to digest the food, as a strong acid, it destroys most bacteria and parasitic life, such as amoeba. These tablets cost little and prevent much suffering.

ULCERATED FUNGUS: see CANDIDA ALBIANS INFECTION.

ULCERS, STOMACH AND DUODENAL: a break in the mucous membrane of stomach or duodenum with loss of surface tissue.

Both gastric (stomach) and duodenal (upper intestines) ulcers can be caused by severe mental and emotional strain and/or nutritional deficiencies. Health problems from them are inevitable. People with ulcers should rest and relax from all pressing worries and problems, then correct their food intake.

Because the stomach and duodenum cannot break down cells, some cooked foods like millet, which is the best, and white rice should be eaten. Both can be served with raw milk, preferably goat's, or a little butter or fruit juice. Lightly steamed vegetables, yogurt, kefir, soured milks if lactose is tolerated, can be eaten. Poi with a touch of butter is very agreeable. Brewer's yeast with the soak water of sprouting buckwheat is excellent to take on an empty stomach between meals. The raw sprouts of buckwheat (see "Sprouting Tables" in *The UNcook Book*, or *Bandwagon to Health*) can be blended in warm water and eaten as porridge. Don't kill this living nutrient with water over 110 degrees or with cooking. Potatoes, yams, squashes, raw bananas and avocado are also excellent if there is no allergy to them.

Avoid raw vegetables and tart fruits until the ulcer heals. Also avoid all fried foods, animal fats, meats, margarine, processed oils, and drinks too hot or too cold.

A good healing treatment for stomach ulcer is raw potato juice. Take one half glass freshly made, several times a day on an empty stomach. Now and then a little raw cabbage juice can be included. Another healing treatment is bee propolis. Suggested dosage: three drops in water three times a day.

We can testify to the immediate relief of duodenal ulcer brought on by raw cabbage juice with a little celery or carrot juice taken on an empty stomach four times a day. Elizabeth can end a flare-up (rare with her now) of duodenal ulcer in three or four days with this soothing remedy. We have the late friend and nutritionist Paavo Airola to thank, and God to praise for His caring love in still guiding us through adversity as well as into the prosperity of health.

URIC ACID: see GOUT.

URINE PROBLEMS (DRIBBLING): inability to control the passing of urine.

Increasingly, more people every year suffer from the annoying, embarrassing and, of late, expensive problem of uncontrollably dribbling urine. Judging from the television advertising that can cost millions of dollars for a single item advertised, the need for an absorbent undergarment must be tremendous. Yet this problem of dribbling may be easily corrected. Sufficient potassium and magnesium, pantothenic acid and vitamin B2 are needed to *control* the passing of urine and also to *pass* urine. Masses of scar tissue in the bladder in older people may decrease its size until much less urine than normal is retained, adding frequent need for voiding to the problem of dribbling, both indicating the need for vitamin E.

Many have been joyously freed of this nagging problem by doing the following: Improve the diet with plenty of the B vitamins in sprouts of all kinds, especially sprouted cereal grains, rice and oat bran, primary yeast, spirulina plankton, bee pollen and fresh wheat germ. Eat two cups of dark leafy green vegetables, preferably raw, a day and fresh fruits for magnesium and potassium. Some people have such deficiencies of these minerals they take up to one gram (1,000 milligrams) of magnesium and up to two grams a day of potassium for awhile. Money spent for protective garments can soon be saved or used to buy more fresh fruits which help to keep from having a dribbling problem.

VAGINITIS: inflammation or infection of the vagina.

One of the most effective discoveries Elizabeth stumbled onto is the ascorbic acid (vitamin C) douche. Our physician helped her establish the amount of Vitamin C to use—a teaspoon full of fine powdered crystal ascorbic acid per pint of lukewarm water. Use all of it. Relief is immediate. Improvement is rapid if douching two to three times a day for an itching, vaginal yeast overgrowth infection. Odor and discharge may soon be eliminated. As improvement comes, the amount of vitamin C may be decreased. Along with douching, she does a vaginal implant made of one-half cup freshly made yogurt to which has been added one tablespoon of L-acidophilus powder. Combine extremely well. This mixture is for the "good" bacterial replacement and for providing growth substance for these bacteria to feed on. At night, insert approximately two teaspoons of the mixture by a syringe with cut off end, a medicine applicator available at drugstores, or even a tampon. Do this five consecutive nights.

Apple cider vinegar also makes a very good douche—four teaspoons to a pint of lukewarm water.

With this treatment, several grams internally of vitamins C and E daily, and an optimal natural diet, a clear vagina and good general health just naturally follow. If you're taking medication, wait until that is over, then do the above treatment. (See also CANDIDA ALBIANS INFECTION.)

VARICOSE VEINS: abnormally swollen or dilated veins.

The more fat deposits (triglycerides) lodged in the veins, the more chance there is for blood clots which cause varicose veins. The best medicine of course is prevention, which means a natural diet with more natural, unsaturated than saturated fats. A widespread problem that results in, among other diseases, varicose veins, is the result of a heavy diet of meat marbled with fat, hydrogenated oils, overheated oils and fats in fried foods and refined carbohydrates which the body converts to sugar for energy and fat storage.

Pliny (60 A.D.) prescribed the powdered root of butcher's broom for healing varicose veins. During the middle ages this herb was cultivated throughout Europe. It resembles asparagus and eaters remained free of circulatory disorders as phlebitis, leg cramps and hemorrhoids. It also gave the eater good energy and vigor. Comfrey tea, root, fresh leaves and shoots, rich in minerals which include the oxygen conserving germanium, and the healing factor alanine have been found to be very helpful in relieving and improving varicose veins.

Vinegar rubs of affected legs, ingesting of one or two teaspoons of vinegar three times a day, vitamin E (up to 1,200 units) and much walking each day help to control and relieve varicose veins. If the sufferer is overweight, he or she should lose weight down to normal.

VITILIGO: white splotches on the skin from depigmentation, at the same time accompanied by dark areas.

Both symptoms of vitiligo are caused by malnutrition from deficiencies. Either the person does not get enough B vitamins in the diet or has a below-par digestive system that does not synthesize them from good carbohydrates in the small intestine.

Vitiligo people either eat poor quality carbohydrates in processed starches from which sufficient B vitamins cannot be synthesized, or they lack sufficient hydrochloric acid for a good digestion that can synthesize B vitamins.

The skin clears when the digestion and the diet are improved greatly with natural sources of the missing vitamins—PABA, pantothenic acid, vitamin C and hydrochloric tablets or capsules. The vitiligo that Elizabeth had slowed down, then mostly cleared when she chose an all-natural diet supplemented with brewer's yeast for B vitamins, green vegetable juice daily and extra vitamin C, primarily to get over Addison's disease. Witnessing the return of natural skin color to all those frightening white spots was a fringe benefit she had not expected. It was one more miracle of healing. (See also FACIAL SIGNS OF SKIN PROBLEMS.)

WARTS: horny growths on the skin, usually on the extremities, commonly caused by a virus.

In all cases of warts it is well to improve the diet before starting a remedy to help get rid of the wart.

There are literally dozens of remedies tried, successful and reported. But what works for one may not work for another. We list here a few of those that have been effective for removing warts for some people we have known. 1) Vitamins E and A rubbed on the wart two or three times a day, or squeezed on an adhesive bandage and placed over the wart. Some say taking 400 to 600 IU of vitamin E and 50,000 to 100,000 units of vitamin A hasten the disappearance of warts. 2) Vitamin C (ascorbic acid) rubbed into the wart after a little olive or castor oil has been applied so the C will stick. Cover with an adhesive bandage. Do daily along with taking one to five grams of vitamin C until wart disappears. Improve the diet. 3) Raw potato, cut and rubbed on several times a day for two or three weeks. 4) Milky juice of fresh, nearly green figs rubbed on several times a day for a week or two. 5) Asparagus, raw, canned or frozen cooked, pureed in blender; eat three or four tablespoons morning and night until warts disappear. 6) Take three to six garlic-parsley tablets a day and/or raw garlic juice on an adhesive bandage and apply before going to bed. This remedy has many followers. 7) Milkweed juice rubbed on two or three times a day is an old Indian remedy. 8) Dandelion root juice rubbed on two or three times a day; Elizabeth just "removed" a small wart of years existence on her ring finger by applying the root juice of healthy, well watered and fed lawn dandelion twice a day. It took just over two weeks. She was amazed and delighted since nothing else was the least bit effective.

WATER BLISTERS: see HERPES, SIMPLEX.

WEIGHT CONTROL: maintaining a certain weight, ideally, a normal one.

The weight problem many people have has many causes. But probably the main causes are underexercising and overeating. In cases of obesity, vitamin E levels are invariably low. Except for rare occurrences of hyperthyroidism and defective metabolism, the main cause of obesity is overeating, experts agree. Nearly half the population of the United States has a weight problem. We are a nation of overfed, undernourished, underexercised people.

Vegetarians, and this includes lacto-vegetarians and ovo-lacto-vegetarians, not only are seldom overweight, they live longer than meat eaters. (They have far less cancer and heart disease. And they have more energy for weight control activity and exercise.) It is difficult to gain weight on a diet made up of lots of vegetables, fruits and moderate amounts of whole grains, nuts, seeds and legumes.

The high meat protein diet advocated in 1872 by a famous physician, and still in vogue, was based on meat from range cattle that had practically no fat. Today it is nearly impossible to buy truly lean meat or fowl. Special feed lots now exist to artificially fatten cattle. Thus it is that the consumer following the high meat and animal protein diet today also gets a diet high in saturated fats, chemicals, estrogens, antibiotics, etc. Considering the fact that half of the proteins we eat can be converted to calories and some ten percent of the fats utilized as calories, we can understand that animal proteins may actually be contributing to overeating and obesity rather than correcting it.

Why does a person gain weight? One reason may be that he or she has a faulty "appestat," caused by food deficiencies that control the appetite. There are other more understandable reasons that have come to light through studies of clinical records of obese patients. For instance, eating two meals a day often brings on weight gain. Larger meals overtax the enzyme producing system which is then unable to utilize much of the food, leaving a large share to be stored as fat. With most Americans eating eighty percent of their food after six P.M., it's easy to understand the nearly universal problem of weight gain. The empty calories of junk foods fail to produce energy. The eater has little "get up and go." He or she gains weight with too many calories and not enough energy to burn them.

Experiments with animals show that on a balanced diet except for thirty-seven percent of the calories coming from fat, the animals soon became obese. Yet many Americans get up to sixty percent of their calories in fats!

Natural foods contain all the nutrients necessary to produce calories for high energy and sustained mental and physical activity. No fat is stored because high energy is conducive to activity, and activity *burns* calories.

Two essential oils called linoleic acid and linolenic acid occurring in fresh seeds, avocado, nuts, and evening primrose oil have been found to help burn fat off the body. A rich source of alpha-linolenic acid has recently been found in black currents, which also have some smaller amount of linoleic acid. Studies in the cases of obese people taking six to eight capsules a day of the natural oil have shown that without altering their diet, weight loss took place in sixty percent of them. The two oils are essential for a number of reasons: they cannot be made from other ingested oils; they are needed for the production of prostaglandins, essential substances that serve as regulators to control many functions in the body; they are effective in the treatment of arthritis, multiple sclerosis and such symptoms of premenstrual syndrome, as breast tenderness and swelling, irritability, abdominal bloating, asthma, weight gain, cramps, backache, joint pains and sugar craving.

Among other problems that evening primrose oil—in conjunction with vitamins B3, B6, C, magnesium and zinc—has relieved, according to studies made at Tulane University, are hypertension and high cholesterol. The best thing about the oil is that it is a natural food with no known adverse side effects.

It's wise to eat all unrefined foods. Make your own mayonnaise out of mashed avocado, seasoned to your taste, or yogurt. Avoid commercial dressings, white flour products, sugar, white rice, etc. There's fiber in natural foods. The more raw things you eat the less you'll gain.

As your diet becomes more nutritious your cravings will become less and less. As they become less you'll not be compelled to overeat. When you don't overeat, you'll feel better. Feeling better, you'll have more energy. With more energy you can start more exercises. The more exercising you do the more pounds you burn off. It's a slow process. But believe us, it's worth the effort.

There's a new wonderful fiber with less calories, a staple in the Japanese diet for centuries. Don't take our word for it. Try it. The name of the fiber is glucomannan. It's the active ingredient in Konjac Root. It can be bought in Japanese stores, with recipes for its use.

Here are some reminders for weight control: it isn't always the amount of food eaten that causes weight gain. It often is the lack of nutrients needed to convert fat to energy. With natural foods, nutrients required for producing energy accompany each calorie; junk foods have few nutrients. They even increase the need for them. There is an axiom here: the more empty calories in junk food eaten, the less energy. The less the energy, the more the compulsion to eat more calories. The result? Eventual obesity.

WHITEHEAD: a small white ball of cholesterol in a pore just under the outer layer of skin, usually appearing on the face.

Whiteheads have been found to result from a vitamin B2 (riboflavin) deficiency.

A middle-aged member of our family, after taking vitamin B2 and an improved diet for a few months found she had no *new* whiteheads. She continued improving her diet and taking vitamin B2 (from yeast) for a year with the whiteheads not disappearing. After she took a daily green drink of mostly leafy vegetables which gave her an abundance of vitamin A along with lots of minerals and other valuable nutrients, plus nuts, seeds and avocado for essential oils necessary for helping to dissolve cholesterol deposits, the whiteheads gradually disappeared. Not only her skin cleared, but most wrinkles disappeared. She felt wonderful.

WORMS: a general term applied not only to pin worms and tapeworms, but amoeba and such parasites as trichomonad and trichinae in undercooked pork—which can grow in and around the vagina, the intestines and the lungs.

Animals fed a diet lacking in sufficient vitamins A, B, B2 and biotin, or folic acid are easily infected with the above parasites and worms. Healthy, optimally fed animals who were even implanted with these parasites did not become infected.

Malnurtured children are more susceptible to worm infestation. Pinworms thrive in the individual whose intake of sugar and refined foods is high. It has been proven by case histories that where worm infestation has been present, an especially nutritious diet, free of processed foods, has been most beneficial to rid the system of worms. Acidophilus culture appears to be particularly beneficial in conquering amoebic dysentery and other infections of the bowels. Stomach acid should be sufficiently high to destroy many parasites harbored in foods. A physician should decide when, if, and how much stomach acid should be taken. The test for it is simple and not expensive. The deficiency in stomach acid can be corrected with betaine hydrochloride or glutamic acid, hydrochloride tablets or capsules bought at the health food store. (See Appendix, Body pH Chart.)

During Elizabeth's childhood, her scrawny little cousin came to spend the summer with them. Elizabeth's mother was horrified when she discovered worms dropped in his pajamas in the morning. She couldn't get him to eat raw garlic, a time-honored folk remedy, but she did put cut slices of the pods in his socks and made him wear his shoes even though it was barefoot season. He passed many more worms that night. Using another remedy handed down from her great-grandmother, Elizabeth was given the task of hulling pumpkin seeds for this small cousin who ate them ravenously. This is now recognized to be effective in expelling worms. She also gave him buttermilk and clabber, the naturally soured, raw milk. With mother's remedies and good, wholesome food, the scrawny cousin gained weight rapidly and returned to his young parents a healthy, happy, little boy, free of worm infestation and full of glowing stories about his Aunt Bessie.

Elizabeth became infected with amoeba in Japan on the way to Sri Lanka where Elton worked for two years. The American Embassy's local doctor prescribed diodoquin which did not rid her of the amoeba. After several months of ill health, Dr. DeSilva, a Sinhalese dentist and neighbor who learned of her problem, chided her for not consulting him. Elizabeth told him she appreciated his concern, but realized he was a dentist and also did not wish to impose on their friendship. Dr. DeSilva scolded Elizabeth more severely than ever saying, "Friendship is helping one another. You go to your friends when in need of help." Showing her to a comfortable chair, he began, "Now you listen to me. From the pattern of your illness, I would say you have the type of infestation that responds best to enterovioform. It's a strong vermifuge but it doesn't take much to help clear the gut of infestation." Having been trained in England first as an M.D. and later taking up dentistry to provide Colombo with a good dentist, he used the British blunt terminology for intestine. "I want you to eat a highly nutritious diet that will protect you from further infestation and restore you to health." The foods he recommended were all fresh, natural, fibrous ones, with no animal protein except an English product called Bosco, a tasty dark brown high protein concoction with the consistency of soft salve. The only cooked foods he allowed were brown rice and steamed or baked potato. He prescribed three glutamic acid hydrochloride tablets after each meal, the tablets Elizabeth had inadvertently left packed with our crated things instead of in our suitcases. You see, she was not taking stomach acid while in Japan and thus became vulnerable to amoeba.

In three days Elizabeth felt well and the fever left. In three weeks she climbed a rock mountain, precipitous and dangerous. She was that strong. It was another great lesson God taught us through error and experience.

XEROSTOMIC: see DRY MOUTH.

ZINC DEFICIENCY: lack of dietary zinc, a trace mineral with many services to perform in the body.

Zinc is needed by every cell in the system. There are many areas of body function, growth, and development in which zinc plays a major role. It is essential for the utilization of protein and the performance of more than thirty enzymes.

Two well known results of zinc deficiency are underdevelopment of sexual organs, especially in boys during puberty, and poor assimilation of vitamin B6 and magnesium. Here is a partial list of other problems for which dietary zinc is needed to bring about improvement or healing:

Acne
Aging
Allergy

Birth defects
Body odor
Cancer
Cracked skin
Dandruff
Diabetes
Dream recall (poor)
Dwarfism
Eczema
Extremities, cold
Facial skin care
Fungus
Growth insufficiency, especially in boys
Hair loss
Healing (slow)
Herpes type II
Itching
Joint problems of knees and hip
Low resistance to infection
Stretch marks
Sexual immaturity especially in boys
Sterility
Subnormal sexual performance
Prostate problems
Rashes
Taste buds (zinc deficiency causes lack of or impaired sense of taste)
Vision problems
Vitamin utilization
Synthesis of Protein
Synthesis of more than thirty enzymes

Foods rich in zinc are oyster, pumpkin seeds, sunflower, flax and sesame seeds, nuts , yeast, green leafy vegetables, eggs and herring. The plant food highest in zinc is pumpkin seeds and the animal food highest in zinc is oysters. Sprouting releases zinc in cereal grains. Some experts believe too much milk, three to six or more cups a day, coupled with zinc deficiency, can stimulate abnormal growth, accounting for so many extra tall young adults in today's world.

Part III

Healthy Weight Control: An Actual Class History

by Elizabeth Baker

In autumn of 1980, Elton was asked to teach a class in weight loss. Since he had booked a trip to Europe with the International College of Applied Nutrition for that time, he suggested I teach the class. We were both into the same research study, lecturing, writing and teaching. The prospective students and their organizer kindly agreed to accept me, and the course was scheduled.

Thirteen ladies enrolled. Their ages ranged from eighteen to seventy, with the majority in their thirties and early forties. They had three things in common: the problem of overweight, anticipation, and enthusiasm. From the moment I saw them I sensed the group made up a very special class.

Imagine having to lose 190 pounds. One lady in the class faced that challenge. The least overweight class member carried some 40 extra pounds. We met once a week in a club house lounge. Sylvia, the spokesperson, an intelligent, warmhearted woman approaching middle age, came for me the first evening.

"We've been told our problem is psychological so many times that we've got real complexes," she laughed. "Yet we're all reasonably happy with our lives, our families, our husbands. It's just ourselves we're unhappy with."

As we drove into the club's parking lot, the other members of the class arrived. Sylvia introduced me while we arranged chairs around a large oblong table. Everybody was on a first name basis. I liked that. I had brought two thermos bottles of herb teas, the first step in getting them off coffee, chocolate, regular tea and soft drinks.

"We're all here to work together for good health through nutrition. Good health is our goal," I said after we settled down around the table. I glanced at each woman. They were a handsome, bright-eyed group. The fact that they had organized themselves some time before, to try to help each other with problems their doctors had considered psychological and/or emotional, meant they were alert, open to suggestion and eager to learn. I agreed with Sylvia who had said on the way over, "They're a pretty terrific bunch of gals."

"What about our problem of being overweight?" asked Ann, one of the largest of the group. She had dark blue eyes and gold hair that glistened under the overhead light.

"The truth about diets is out," I told them. "Special dieting and *permanent* weight loss simply do not go together. After all the countless books and articles written on dieting, it is becoming evident that overweight has as its cause the dysfunction of two hormones.

"We know that each body function is governed by hormones. The two that regulate weight are *prostaglandin*, which balances fat storage in normal quantities, and *somatotropin* which stimulates muscle growth as it burns fat and releases energy. Overweight people often lack normal energy. Their muscle size is small. Both muscle size and power decrease as weight increases. Fat is not burned off. All this because they lack the two hormones in sufficient quantity and quality."

Sylvia's hand raised and I nodded at her. "How do we correct such deficiencies?"

I could understand her skepticism. She was one who had tried various "diets" to lose weight, only to gain back more than ever.

"The amino acids lysine, tryptophan, ornithine and arginine make up somatotropin. When we eat these nutrients our body makes plenty of that fat-burning hormone. With the burning of fat, energy is released and muscles grow. In other words, not only is our fat burned, we have more energy and stronger muscles to manipulate our bodies and increase our activity.

"Experts are finding weight is lost only when sufficient hormones are present to stimulate cells to convert fat."

"And what gives us sufficient hormones to stimulate those cells to convert fat?" Ann put in as I paused.

"A wide range of foods give tryptophan, lysine, arganine and ornithine—seeds, nuts, whole grains, legumes, chicken, turkey, fish, eggs—all-natural foods that haven't lost nutrients in processing. In this case, chiefly amino acids. A number of researchers of obesity contend overweight people may need to eat a little animal protein except red meat, for sufficient weight regulating factors. As to what foods contain specific amino acids, I suggest you get *The Nutrition Almanac* available at health food stores, and study the tables on the essential amino acids and those on food composition.

"There is yet another hormone that some research physicians feel destroys fat. It is called HGH or simply GH. They say it increases muscle and burns fat. They also believe, although regular exercise is beneficial, switching to a natural nutrition program of fifty percent or over of raw foods is the all-important decision to make in weight control. Once into and maintaining that program, they warn, people should expect to lose *very* slowly for the first month or two while the body is adjusting. They add a postscript: throw out old bad habits like smoking, alcohol, drugs, coffee and tea.

"Lastly, they give a word of warning: some weight loss programs (appetite depressors, protein powders, concentrated pill foods) may alert the body to protect itself against starvation by conserving and storing fat. This earmarking of every possible calorie for eventual storage translates to quick, steady weight gain on the already overweight person.

"A little later we'll discuss and plan a nutrition program for each of you. For now, we'll discuss health or the lack of it." I could see all sorts of physical ills in their faces, the color and condition of their skin, their fingernails, the way they sat. There wasn't a truly healthy one in the class.

I recalled the many times doctors had told me my problem was nerves. I thought of many friends in the United States who had been told the same, then given tranquilizers, mood elevators, sleeping pills. And I thought of friends in Mexico where we spend our winters. They had all, sooner or later, discussed their health problems with me. Health is of deepest concern to those who don't have it. Tragically, that includes just about every adult. Without exception, they had each been told by their doctors that their problems were mainly nerves!

"We will concentrate on health first. The healthy person is not obese." A murmur of relief swept the room. The girls, as I affectionately thought of them, smiled, chatted with newly found freedom from the guilt/blame syndrome and urged me to continue. They were curious as to what illness I thought I could see at little more than a glance at them.

"It's no secret at all," I began. "You can see it as well as anyone else. Most of you have puffs around or under your eyes—water retention that could indicate a kidney problem."

With few exceptions they pounced on the last statement, telling me of living with persistent, annoying and serious edema. Most of them had taken or were taking diuretic pills.

As they quieted, I went on. "At least two of you, Sylvia and Matilda, may have a thyroid problem. The eyeballs protrude."

"Yes, that's true," they said.

"Betty, Andrea, and especially Dottie and Hilda probably have menstruation cramps, get car or sea sick, may be troubled with burning lips, sometimes sore mouths, and anemia."

"That's right. That's what happens to me," two said.

"Now tell us what reveals this to you," said Betty, a handsome forty-year-old so large we had to find a special chair for her.

"The iris of your eyes floats above the lower lids. There's white showing between the blue, gray or brown part of the eye, and the lower lids when you look straight in front of you. It's what the Japanese call *sam paku*. And some of you don't have a good color tone to your faces."

Out came the little mirrors I had told Sylvia to have each one bring.

"What causes the eyes to 'float' like that?" Esther asked.

"Mainly lack of vitamin B6, say the experts," I replied.

"I'm going right out and buy some," Dottie put in.

"If you decide to take a B6 supplement, be sure you are getting all the other B vitamins in foods. You could throw your vitamin intake off balance. Remember we can't repair our bodies with one vitamin any more than we can repair a run-down house with just a new door. We have to have several or many repair materials—lumber, nails, paint, plaster. Nutrients, in our case."

"What else do you see, Elizabeth?" asked Matilda, an ample, grandmotherly matron.

"According to an outstanding allergist my husband knows, people whose ears tip out at the top, away from the head, have allergy tendencies. If that is true, and we have observed it is with many people, some of you may be allergy prone."

"Our family has a lot of allergies," volunteered Flo, a fair-skinned, light-haired, comely young mother. "My husband and children have prominent ears."

"People with fine blond hair also are allergy prone."

"That must be right," Flo went on. "I'm plagued with

allergies, but our doctor has always felt it was all in my mind."

"What about our complexions? What do they show?" Connie asked. She was an elderly woman, still beautiful, with black eyes and white hair. Her light skin was marred by white, pigmentless patches on her neck and lower part of her face.

"Skin eruptions may have as many causes as victims. Our nutrition-minded physician, Dr. Silver, has found that when the diet of most such people is improved, the skin clears, whether of acne, rashes, eczema, brown spots from adrenal exhaustion, or white patches, called vitiligo. In such cases there's usually a severe deficiency of most if not all the vitamins known, especially the B vitamins and vitamins A and C.

"While we 're still on the subject of skin, let's look at everyone. A pale, colorless skin usually suggests anemia. A grayish white skin may indicate an unhealthy condition of some kind, like cancer. A pasty, yellowish white might suggest liver and intestinal problems. A yellow skin, definitely liver-gall bladder."

"My daughter is a pasty, sallow color. She eats a steady diet of hamburger, French fries, cokes and pizza. Her boy friend cooks at a hamburger pizza place," Hilda said when I paused.

Her statement brought on a hum of comments about family members or acquaintances with similar diets, sallow skin and ill health.

Suddenly I was overwhelmed with the fact that the majority of people, whether old or young, show signs of deficiencies, of lack of proper development of bone structure, of ill health. I recalled all too clearly Dr. Munger, when baffled by the cause of my woeful lack of energy and resistance to respiratory infections, saying in annoyance, "We all live with something, Elizabeth."

Since then I've thought many times, it doesn't have to be. Most people could be healthy if only they ate natural foods, drank pure water, and did not indulge in the things that brought poisons into their bodies, such as drugs, tobacco, alcohol and the chemicals in processed foods.

"Fingernails tell quite a story," I picked up again, trying to keep focused. "Thank you for leaving off nail polish for tonight. Brittle fingernails that split and break or are very thin, indicate malnutrition, a lack of vitamin A, protein, or B12. White spots or opaque, milky nails may show zinc deficiency. Nails that are flat and curl down over the ends of the fingers may indicate high blood pressure (hypertension). And the reverse, or saucer-shaped ones that turn slightly up, may show low blood pressure from adrenal exhaustion or loss of salt in the urine. I had saucer fingernails for many years.

"Ridges can be caused by lack of cobalamin (B12). These ridges sometimes show up during the menstruation period, probably indicating a vitamin B6 and zinc deficiency. Horizontal ridges, which usually go with brittle nails, can be caused by anemia, nervousness, malnutrition. I was anemic all my life. I took bottles of Lugol solution, iron pills and liver shots with no noticeable results. Since eating all-natural foods which includes chlorella, a new name for fresh water algae (spirulina plankton), I have an excellent blood count. All those pills and shots were wasted on me. I could have been killed from iron build up from shots one doctor gave me over a period of years.

"When the nails grow away from the quick it's usually because of a fungus. When the diet contains adequate B vitamins the nails gradually grow back as the fungus disappears. Fungus thrives only in an unhealthy, poorly nourished body. That's been a problem I've battled off and on for years. My last escapade with a bad food which caused diarrhea and a forced fast, showed up, among other places, in my nails. They've almost grown back, but here's one that still has a way to go yet." I extended the third finger of my left hand for them to see. It was the one that had always been the most affected by deficiencies of every kind, making it from time to time, thinnest, the most brittle and having the most ridges.

"While you're holding the mirrors, let's have a look at tongues." I dug a compact out of my purse, stuck out my tongue and studied it, something I hadn't done for months. I was delighted to see no white coating on it, a rare condition for me, in times past.

"If your tongue is coated over with a thick, velvetlike layer of white, you have bad bacteria in the intestines and putrefactive stools."

Most everyone had a white coating on the tongue. Ann had none, the only one completely free of it.

"Mine is a nice red," she said, smiling in triumph.

"Mine is coated, but around the edges it's redder than yours," Esther laughed. A jolly, fun-loving, prematurely grayed woman, she stuck her tongue out for all of us to see.

I had never seen a more brilliantly red tongue. I explained the experts say it is probably caused by a niacin (B3) deficiency, that niacin was essential for the normal function of the brain, the nervous system and the circulation. I refrained from saying that massive doses have proven very effective in the treatment of schizophrenia.

I held my breath for Esther. She had told me that for two years she had taken the anticoagulant Coumadin, a drug very harmful to the digestive system which inhibits the synthesis of the B vitamins in the intestines.

I hadn't expected to discuss individual tongues. Without looking at anyone, I went on to explain, first, that a normal tongue is an even, pinkish red color without any cracks or fissures, and smooth without being shiny. When someone suffers a vitamin B complex deficiency for an extended time, as in the case of taking almost any kind of drug, especially The Pill, taste buds clump together and the grooves and indentation known as geographic tongue, form. Teeth marks along the sides appear when the tongue becomes enlarged or beefy from a lack of pantothenic acid.

"This fat tongue condition was so pronounced at one period during my illness that my tongue was chewed up along the sides from getting in the way of my teeth. A magenta or purplish tongue often indicates a B2 deficiency."

"My tongue tells me I may not be very healthy. Do you want to take me next?" Ann asked.

"Of course, Ann."

She leaned her plump torso forward, elbows on the table. "I've always thought of myself as being healthy, ignoring little things like hemorrhoids, constipation and bleeding polyps. The doctor is insisting I have surgery but with two small children and no money, I can't. Anyway, I read an article saying if you eat right they'll shrink and not bother any more. Is that true?"

"With qualifications, yes. In places in the world where no refined foods are eaten, hemorrhoids, polyps and constipation are practically unknown."

"Why is that? Because they eat bulky foods?"

"Probably the main reason. Other reasons may be chemicals, artificial foods, insecticides, polluted water and air, even inorganically fertilized food crops."

"It sounds grim. Do we have much of a chance?" Ann was dead serious.

"Yes we do," I said. For assurance I told her about having the

same problems—constipation, hemorrhoids and polyps. Before
we could afford surgery for me, my husband's career took him to
underdeveloped countries where there was little processed food.
We lived off the country and my health improved. However, not
until years later when I got on all-raw foods and extra
magnesium, did hemorrhoids and polyps shrink and constipation end.

"Are they gone forever?"

"Go back on a conventional diet and they may return. I
learned the hard way."

Ann went on to say she and her sister, during high school and
college, gorged on sweets as they studied every night. "Two of us
still go on sugar binges once in a while," she confessed. "We're
as compulsive as alcoholics. We're real sugar addicts."

"Most of us are," I assured her. "At birth we're started on
formulas containing sugar. By the time we're a year or two old,
we're hooked. But there's a way to end our craving. We'll get to
that soon.

"For now, try to eat only natural, untreated, unsprayed foods.
Take no sugar—only a little honey if you have to. No coffee, tea,
alcohol, or tobacco. No processed foods like white flour, white
rice, pastas, canned foods, crackers, and so on."

"Ad nauseam," Betty said. She laughed but there was sadness
in her large, round face.

I studied the faces of this intensely interested, highly
motivated class of women. There were many signs of premature
aging, of unfortunate body changes like graying and dull, brittle
hair; vertical wrinkles or "whistle" marks on the lips; (lack of
pantothenic acid, linoleic acid, folacin and/or vitamins B6 and
B2 respectively). Some of them had premature wrinkling of the
face; hair on the upper lip (lack of estrogen); red "turkey" neck
(too much sugar and/or alcohol); bad posture, especially as
manifested by the dowager's hump, even on one twenty-eight-
year old; "liver" spots on face and hands. Stretch marks (lack of
zinc) zigzagged the bare shoulders of Hilda, as she sat in a
sleeveless mumu.

I could have wept for these victims of our so-called civilized
way of life. Controlling my emotion, I went over to the serving
bar.

"I've two kinds of tea for you to try. One is slippery elm. The
other is comfrey from my own garden. They're both very
special, although you may not like them." I smiled, even though

my heart cried in sympathy for these wonderful women starting on the long, rocky road to health and a slender figure.

The second session found my girls and me again seated around the table of the club lounge. I had decided against the brief, fact-packed, opening lecture. These women had not enrolled in the course to learn a lot of general information. They were there to find out how each could help herself.

"Because you all showed such interest in the study of health—or lack of it—as applied to you, we are going to take up your problems individually." A wave of approval passed around the table. "Betty, would you like to be first?" I chose the big beautiful 340 pounder because she was outgoing, friendly, and because she rubbed her shoulders frequently in an effort to relieve pain.

"Yes. Oh, I *hoped* you'd start with me. I've so many questions." Her melodious voice rang with eagerness. "Today I examined my tongue in sunlight. Do you know it has nearly all the symptoms you told us about last week? My bright red tongue I thought was so healthy shows a niacin deficiency. I want to know what to do about that, but first I'd like to know about my arthritis. I read an article in the paper the other day by a doctor. He says there is no cure for arthritis."

"Many contend there is no cure. If they are referring to cures from medicines, they are right," I said. "But a number of physicians have found that we get arthritis from the foods we eat, from the way we live. And we get over it the same way, although with different foods and a modified manner of living."

"What foods give us arthritis and what foods get us over it?"

"In my case, the pain of arthritis left a few days after quitting sugar," I told them.

"I've just finished reading *Sugar Blues*. I'm so convinced I shouldn't eat sugar, I almost quit."

"Then you've taken the first step toward getting over arthritis."

"How bad was your arthritis, Elizabeth?"

"Bad enough to knot my finger joints. I had to give up guitar and knew I'd soon have to quit playing the piano and typing. I had painful calcium deposits on my elbows and on three vertebrae of the lower back, injured a long time ago. I lived for years with lower back pain, partly from the calcium deposits there."

"What were you told to do about them? I also have calcium

deposits." piped up Sylvia.

"One doctor told me not to eat high calcium foods. Yet not long after that another doctor found that my serum level of calcium was very low. I had osteoporosis. Something was causing the calcium to be taken from the bones and deposited on the joints," I said.

"That's what's happening to me and I have constant pain. In my hands, my elbows. But the worst is in my shoulders. I can't raise my arms higher than this." She extended her hands, then lifted her arms no more than a few inches above the table, writhing with pain with even that elevation. "How and when did you get the calcium out of the deposits and back in your bones?" Her great bulk bounced with laughter from her joke.

"After the fast when I found what I was allergic to and ate only the natural foods that agreed with me, the arthritis, even the deposits, gradually disappeared."

"What were those foods?" Sylvia queried.

"Most fruits and vegetables I could eat, especially the leafy green vegetables. At that time my best starches were whole grain rice, corn and millet. Since then I've gone to sprouted cereal grains and buckwheat, eaten whole and raw at breakfast, or blended to a cream, dropped in cracker-size dabs on plastic wrap and dehydrated at 100 degrees into delicious raw crackers. I eat no meat. Experts have found arthritics should avoid animal proteins. The incidence of arthritis among meat eaters is great, while vegetarians seldom have arthritis."

"I've read that most of us eat too much meat."

"Biochemists, nutritionists and many doctors are convinced that is true. Especially people in America eat too much red meat. They eat twice as much beef, lamb and pork now as they did before the Second World War. It's become the fashion and is far overstressed by restaurants, the industry and reducing diets. The incidence of both arthritis and cancer have risen proportionately with the rise in meat consumption. Whether or not it's principally meat that's responsible for arthritis remains to be proven. Many nutritionally oriented doctors who have helped patients get over arthritis contend there are additional factors besides beef and other animal proteins contributing to the great increase in arthritis. Table sugar and refined white flour, for instance. In my case, especially since I was a light meat eater, leaving refined carbohydrates entirely out of my diet started immediate improvement in arthritis. Leaving off allergy foods finished the process."

"But I have ulcers and diabetes."

"Do you take insulin?"

"At the moment, no. I have. But since I was borderline, my new doctor is having me control it with diet."

"That's great."

"Because the doctors allow it, I've been eating some sugar, although I know now I don't need to. And white bread and meat. Meat doesn't bother the ulcers. I eat a lot of all kinds, but mainly beef. I've always thought, too, that I would lose weight by eating meat."

"Meat has a lot of calories," I pointed out.

"It does? Then what should I eat?" they wanted to know.

"Green leafy vegetables which have some protein, are full of vitamins and minerals and very low in calories. When you leave off meat, especially of the red muscle variety, you leave off hard, saturated fat. And you don't need that. Include a tablespoon of polyunsaturated oil a day, which you do need. A crude, raw, unprocessed oil like corn oil, or safflower oil, or sesame, or sunflower or olive oil. Grocery stores are beginning to stock the crude peanut oil. So far you have to go to a health food store for the others. Don't buy any oil unless it says on the label, 'No preservatives, no solvents.' Some oil labels say 'No preservatives' but they have had the flavor, the color and sediment taken out by solvents—petroleum products. And solvents can't be entirely separated from the oils. They give some of us a very bad time because they still contain some toxicity from the processing."

"Thanks, Elizabeth. I've a headful of things I can do for myself. What should I do about B3 deficiency?"

"Take primary yeast, a bulk brand. Start with a teaspoon at meals and work up to a rounded tablespoon. Take it in water or juice. And your diabetes just may disappear with the living foods I'll help you plan."

Several in the class were still taking notes when we moved on to the next person. It flashed across my mind that we had hardly said a word about weight, and Betty was the most obese person present. The pressing problems to her were not so much obesity as the arthritis, ulcers and diabetes she suffered. Of course her excess weight contributed to those ills. But the noteworthy fact was that although she had come to the class primarily to learn how to lose weight, she was more interested in learning how to eat right for improving her health. The pounds would naturally start coming off with that diet.

"Flo, would you like to be next?"

"Yes, but I don't have problems you can put your finger on, like Betty's"

"What do you mean?"

"Well, my doctor can't find anything wrong with me except that I'm overweight some 50 pounds. And that's because I'm a compulsive eater."

"You're convinced of that?"

"I can't come up with a better answer. He says it's psychological. That I'm bored because I'm tied to the four-month-old baby I'm nursing."

"Do you agree?"

"No, I don't. It's true I was unhappy when I found I was pregnant. We have a boy nine and a seven-year-old girl, an ideal family, we thought. But we're all four enjoying this baby immensely. I just don't feel good. I can hardly get up of a morning, I'm so tired. I suppose it's because I wake up about four o'clock and can't go back to sleep. My heart pounds, my legs feel creepy-crawly and I've a headache."

"Are you hungry when you get up?"

"I'm empty. My stomach's a vacuum. But I'm not really hungry. When I eat, however, I want more and more food. I crave sweets."

Ann's hand went up at the same time she spoke out. "Flo, haven't you read *Sugar Blues* yet?"

Nadine's hand shot up for attention. "Flo and I bought the book together. She hasn't read it yet because my husband's reading it. I'll get it to her tomorrow."

"I know I shouldn't eat sugar but so far I haven't been able to quit," Flo went on. She tilted her head and looked at me with the appealing eyes of a child in distress. "I get a real lift from candy bars. I've so much to do, what with the baby and all. But the . . . "

"You get a letdown and a headache?"

"Yes. And then I'm depressed. My doctor's even given me mood elevators."

"Did they work?"

"They got me so hopped up I think I would have committed murder if I'd kept on taking them. But I quit at the end of the first day. I didn't sleep any for two nights. I thought I'd go crazy."

How my heart reached out to this lovely, twenty-nine-year-old wife and mother. She had much the same experience that I had had with a mood elevator called Elavil.

I recalled feeling excited after taking the first tablet at breakfast, but didn't associate the feeling with the drug. After the next one I felt irritated but attributed the feeling to fast pulse after eating. But after taking the third Elavil tablet, I knew the drug was the cause of my pounding heart, my severe, intense determination to vent my vile feelings on someone. I was rational enough to warn Elton to keep everyone away from me, to give me some yogurt and help me to bed.

"I feel evil," I remember saying as I looked around for something to hurl crashing through the window. "Oh God! Don't let me do anything violent."

Elton had kept silent. He knew I would do nothing drastic. I was as weak and limp as wilted lettuce.

I looked up at Flo. "I've known of just such a reaction."

"Then you don't think it was partly psychological?"

"Not one bit. You might ask your doctor about a glucose tolerance test and serum mineral test. When the results come back to him, be sure you get copies."

"I will. And I'll show them to you. But until then, is there anything I can do?"

"Leave off all sugar, white flour, white rice, tea, coffee and *all* processed foods. Take chromium tablets, the maximum dosage suggested on the bottle. Do you think you can do that?"

"I'll try. I just hope I don't start craving sweets."

"Some nutrition-minded physicians suggest drinking a glass or two of water, then eating a sweet fruit: bananas, papaya, apples or raisins. But try very hard to eat a small helping of fish or chicken or nuts or seeds every day along with lots of vegetables, especially the..."

"Green leafy ones," she finished, laughing.

"It's my turn," said Ann after our ten minute break in which I served spearmint and camomile tea from our garden. Mother of two sturdy boys, she was at thirty-two, attractive in spite of 116 pounds too many for her medium height and fine bones. Like so many overweight people, she presented to the world a bright happy countenance. Her conversation was animated and cheerful, her sense of humor enviable, her laughter frequent and contagious.

"Except for anemia, I'm healthy as a wild moose. And just as heavy. I'm never sick. My one problem is my voracious appetite. I quit sugar twenty-seven days ago. But now I'll cook a pot of baked beans and eat them all. Or a big pizza. Or a meatloaf or a whole fried chicken. Some days I can keep from eating all day. But then I'll start with a few nibbles of cheese or lunch meat and keep on eating until midnight."

Obviously Ann was a real food addict. I took note of the braces on her teeth, crooked from prenatal deficiencies that allowed the tooth arches of her mouth to be narrow and under-developed. I saw white spots on her fingernails—zinc deficiency which could account for her anemia and colorless hair.

As she talked we learned that her problems included blood pressure of 186/110. She also had claustrophobia and short periods of depression.

"Have you noticed any incidence of either since you stopped eating sugar?" I asked. Claustrophobia, a notable symptom of hypoglycemia, had troubled me for years before I learned the cause. It, along with bad dreams and nightmares, had disappeared when I quit eating refined sugar.

"Come to think of it, I haven't. Does sugar cause that?"

"For lots of us. How about nightmares?"

"I haven't had any lately. But sometimes I still have troublesome dreams. Does hypoglycemia cause them too?"

"With myself and others I've known and read about, disturbing dreams often accompany hypoglycemia, even though a person is off sugar. Some allergy to food, chemicals, toxic odors like car fumes, polyester or hot asphalt, can trigger low blood sugar. After such exposure, I usually have tense, disturbing dreams."

"What can I do right now? I want to start immediately to conquer my appetite."

"Have you thought of a hair analysis and blood tests to determine your mineral levels?"

"Yes. I can have that done soon. Do you have some quick suggestions for good general diet for me now?"

I smiled to myself. Everyone wants a good diet planned *on request*. But that may not be possible. Each person is different and has individual needs; perhaps allergies and sensitivities, especially at first.

I thought of Ann's comment about what she gorged on. The foods she mentioned were all high proteins, mostly containing red muscle meats. I wondered if, like so many obese people, she had been advised not to eat any whole grain breads or cereals because of their caloric content. Such advise almost invariably leads to B vitamin deficiency, among other adverse conditions. It would take a lot more knowledge of Ann's case, and an hour or so to work out a diet specifically for her. She soon realized what she had asked me to do and suggested she see me later.

"In the meantime, Ann, try to eat lots of vegetables and no muscle meat. A little fish or chicken instead. And vegetables that grow above ground. You might try eating frequent small meals. Some people lose weight only in that manner. It's called the nibble diet."

Sylvia, the spokesperson for the group, and I had already talked of her problems—constant headache, hemorrhoids from too hard a stool (constipation), cysts the size of pop bottle lids all over her body, compulsive eating, and many food allergies. She had asked for the name and address of the allergist, Dr. Elsie Mooreburn. Before the class started, she had made an appointment to see her.

Nadine, three months pregnant with her second baby, had consulted me a few days before to discuss a prenatal diet that took into consideration acetone in the urine, an allergy to wheat and most grains, and her weight problem.

Dottie, a friend of mine and already a patient of Dr. Mooreburn, had recently made much progress toward health by finding some of her countless food and chemical allergies. A lot of her overweight problem had been water retention, which had disappeared when she avoided the allergens and ate naturally diuretic foods such as asparagus and watermelon. Having already lost nearly 20 pounds, she joined the class anyway to learn nutrition-oriented ways to health and more resistance to allergies.

"You spoke of a hair analysis some time ago, Dottie. Did you have one?"

"Not yet. I've an appointment for tomorrow."

"What's a hair analysis?" asked another class member.

" A one ounce sample of hair one and one half inches long from the scalp out, is snipped from the lower back part of the head. It is analyzed for mineral content. In the hands of an experienced, nutrition-oriented physician, such an analysis, coordinated with a blood analysis, can cast a lot of light on a patient's mineral assimilation, deficiencies and excesses of both essential and toxic minerals."

"Have researchers found a correlation between mineral deficiencies and allergies?" Dottie asked.

"Yes. There's a synergistic action between them and other nutrients. Normally, the intestines manufacture the B vitamins from food. The body synthesizes vitamin D from sunshine and vitamin A from the precursor, beta carotene, found in yellow, orange and dark green vegetables and fruits. But the body appears not to be able to synthesize minerals. They all have to come from foods and/or the water we drink. Many minerals are lost in food processing and in cooking, especially when the water they are cooked in is poured down the sink drain. A lot of people, including restaurant cooks and chefs, feed the sink better than they do themselves and their customers."

"What are some of the symptoms of deficiencies?"

"They are legion. I'll mention only a few mineral deficiencies. One of the most widespread deficiencies is calcium, manifested in osteoporousis, or porous bones. During the Korean War it was found to be widespread among the young soldiers."

"Isn't that a condition of older people? And doesn't it have to start somewhere along one's life?"

"Not according to anthropologists, biochemists, and some physicians. Among wild animals, the opposite holds true. The older the animal, the denser the bones. Scrimshaw artists and bone carvers choose the bones of older animals because they are finer and harder."

"Is food processing the reason we don't get enough calcium?" one woman questioned.

"It may be only part of the cause. Sufficient magnesium has to be present for calcium to be utilized properly. There has to be a balance between calcium and magnesium. Experts say about two parts calcium to approximately one part magnesium, but some people need a greater proportion of magnesium. I for one. There should be sufficient minerals in the soil for good growth of the plants we eat."

"Is that the main function of magnesium? Helping calcium to be assimilated?"

"That's only one of its many functions. Magnesium is necessary for muscle cells. For good function of all muscles— heart, intestines and so on. Muscle cramps, muscle spasms, and charley horses, may occur when there is a magnesium deficiency. Magnesium helps the muscles to relax. It's very important to the heart, a large muscle. It also must be present for vitamin B6 to be utilized."

"We're convinced, Elizabeth. Thank you," the class assured me.

Janie raised her hand to be heard. "May I be next? I have spasms all the time in the muscles of my back, in my diaphragm, sometimes in my face, my eyelids, my arms. Charley horses so bad I've sometimes had to walk with crutches. My doctor says I should quit nursing my new baby, but I don't want to. The doctor seems to think the spasms and cramps will get better if I do. They aren't as bad as they were during pregnancy. At times then I couldn't even walk."

"Have you had blood tests to learn what your serum levels of calcium-magnesium, potassium-sodium are?"

"Only for calcium after my doctor had me take megadoses of calcium for a year. When I started having severe headaches, he took a blood test for calcium. The serum level was way above high normal. If I took magnesium, would it help me with the spasms, the muscle cramps, the fatigue that I've lived with for well over a year?"

"It's helped lots of people. It helped me get over muscle spasms and cramps, constipation and insomnia." I hesitated a moment, looking at this young woman. I had never heard of anyone having such widespread muscle spasms and cramps. My thoughts were flooded with memories of awakening from sleep by such painful leg muscle cramps I could not walk or even stand, cramps that made me cry out with severe pain. When I reported the excruciating distress, the annoying eye twitches, the creeping muscle spasms across my lower rib cage, our conventional doctor gave me pain pills and muscle relaxers. They made me listless, irritable, nauseous.

"What did you do for muscle spasms?" she asked.

"At first I took dolomite, one third teaspoon three times a day. I had read a great deal about it. Many doctors and biochemists in the 1960's and early 1970's thought that dolomite, a natural mineral substance, contained the ideal balance of calcium and magnesium. In addition to dolomite, I took three tablets a day of magnesium oxide. Both dolomite and magnesium oxide with meals. The muscle cramps, the spasms, the eyelid twitching disappeared in about a week.

"A year after that Dr. Silver, our new nutrition-minded

physician, prescribed the first hair analysis. I was found to have nearly normal levels of magnesium and calcium, potassium and sodium, but dangerously high levels of mercury and lead. He had me put in the hospital where he gave me the intravenous chelating agent E.D.T.A. That lowered the mercury and lead levels effectively but it also drastically lowered the serum levels of zinc, manganese, magnesium and calcium. Soon after he found me to be osteoporotic.

"I got the muscle spasms and charley horses back again. I was consulting Dr. Mooreburn, the allergist, at the time and she suggested two teaspoons of calcium citrate and one half teaspoon of plain milk of magnesia with each meal for a week, then one third teaspoon thereafter. The spasms were better after one day and the charley horses stopped after two. It was a miracle."

Janie was taking notes. When she finished, she looked up with her face full of hope. "I've quit taking calcium. I only need to take magnesium, and I have a big bottle of it. I'll start right in tonight. If it worked for you, it might well work for me. Oh, I hope. I hope."

"I do too, Janie."

"Shall we continue on around the table from where we left off last class? I asked after everyone sat down the next week.

Matilda, a quiet, plump woman in her mid sixties, put up her hand and smiled with expectation. Her eyes had the distressed liver, fatigued look, and her eyeballs protruded as though from thyroid trouble. Her colorless skin suggested anemia. There was puffiness around her eyes, ankles and hands. Her breath had the peculiar odor so often encountered in older people who lack sufficient hydrochloric acid (stomach acid) to digest their food well.

"Please do continue," she said in her low, slow voice. "I'm next. I have so many things wrong I don't know where to start."

"High blood pressure?" It was a logical question, what with her obesity and rapid breath.

"Yes, I don't know how high but the doctor shakes his head when he takes it. He just says for me to continue to take the Ser-Ap-Es he prescribes."

"Has he suggested a diet for you?"

"Not really. But he did tell me to avoid pastries and animal fats."

"Do you?"

"Not as much as I should. My husband's mother was from Florence, Italy. She was famous for her cooking. My husband's hobby is making all the fancy desserts, pastries, muffins that she taught him. He's overweight, too, and has a heart condition."

Many people, just like Matilda and her husband, live to eat. By mid life most all of them have degenerative illnesses, victims of artificial, and overcooked, processed, nutrition-robbed, additive-poisoned foods. The same effort, the same creativity in food preparation and serving could have been expended on natural foods, unharmed with additives and depletion. They would have given health instead of disease.

"It's very difficult to lower blood pressure without eliminating, as your doctor says, all pastries first of all, and most hard fats. There are gourmet cookbooks available based on natural foods, with emphasis on fresh fruits and vegetables, nuts, seeds and whole grains, no hard fats and no sugar. Then of course there's *The UNcook Book* which Elton and I authored."

"But how can you make desserts without sugar? Do you advocate using artificial sweeteners?"

"I'll answer your second question first. Since my chemist husband's recent review of modern biochemistry, we've been convinced that nothing artificial should be ingested, including sweeteners. Saccharin is carcenogenic and evidence shows aspartame (NutraSweet) may cause brain damage. Artificial substances—chemicals—are all toxic, mildly, moderately or severely. The liver, our main detoxifying organ, has to reduce them to simpler compounds and the kidneys have to eliminate the resulting garbage. Some toxic compounds are also thrown off by the lungs, the skin and the intestines. This is all additional unnecessary work, over and above the call of duty for these organs of the body. Overwork means added stress. Over a period of time, one or all of these organs may break down. Then we begin to find problems such as liver damage (far more widespread than is generally thought), kidney failure, digestive malfunction, respiratory diseases and skin disorders, to mention some.

Matilda and the rest sat quiet and attentive.

"Now for your first question. I've been working on recipes for a book of no-sugar, no-artificial-sweetener desserts. It's a fun project, but slow. I started by making a list of natural sweets—raisins, dates, date sugar (finely ground hard dates), honey, barley syrup, sweet rice flower and syrup, carob, maple sugar and syrup, black strap molasses and figs. From those sweeteners are coming my dessert recipes. There are, of course, many sweet fruits such as bananas, blueberries, papaya, honey dew and watermelon. I rarely make dessert for us or our company. We eat fresh fruit for dessert. If we crave something really sweet, and that doesn't often happen, we eat peeled, frozen bananas (sweeter tasting because freezing breaks down the cells), dates, or any fruit dried the unsulfured way."

"What about calories? I thought all those sweet fruits were loaded with calories."

"They are, compared to asparagus, tomatoes, leaf lettuce or cantaloupe. But compared to cookies, or pie, cake, dessert crepes or mousses and puddings, they are low.

"Take, for instance, chocolate brownies. One hundred grams (two squares) have 486 calories; 100 grams of banana (a medium sized one), eighty-five calories; one hundred grams of cantaloupe (one quarter melon), thirty calories. Even dates, a very high calorie fruit, have only 270 calories in 100 grams (about ten dates). The same number of grams of butter cookies, oatmeal or chocolate cookies, or plain vanilla wafers have over 400 calories. I've seen many people not hesitate to take two or three cookies yet use strict control in eating dates or nuts because, 'They're so fattening.' Yet the dates and nuts have half the calories and from five to twenty times more vitamins and minerals than equal their weight in most cookies. "

"I've always thought I was overweight because of a thyroid problem. What you are saying is, it's all calories."

"Problems of health and weight may be caused by a combination of factors. It is true that a hypothyroid condition can contribute to obesity. The gland does not produce enough thyroxine to burn enough calories.

"On the other hand, excess weight can accumulate from these caloric-producing substances—table sugar, refined white flour (starch), animal fats, vegetable oils, animal protein, sweet fruits and vegetable protein and so on—in about that order."

"Are you saying proteins have calories?"

"Yes. Complete proteins—those containing the eight or so essential amino acids for the adult, nine for children, are needed for maintenance and repair. Any excess has to be converted to calories to be burned as energy or stored as fat. In this conversion of excess protein to calories, an excess of ammonia and uric acid is produced, substances the kidneys have to work overtime to throw off."

"What you're saying is that eating too much meat is bad two ways. It overtaxes the kidneys and makes a person put on weight."

"Exactly, especially if that person doesn't do exercise to utilize those extra calories as energy."

"You stress eating high fiber foods and raw foods. I have colitis and must stay on a bland diet."

"A bland diet can be a high fiber one. Eat mainly slightly cooked or raw vegetables and fruits. Puree them if necessary. However, I favor pureeing your food in your mouth. Masticate thoroughly, chewing each bite from forty to a hundred times. Pureeing the food in your mouth thoroughly mixes it with saliva. You see, approximately one third of the digestion of food takes place in the mouth."

"I realize I lose a lot of nutrition in cooking."

"Yes, an average of about fifty percent. But if you eat only unrefined, unprocessed foods you may get ample nutrition providing you eat a great variety of vegetables and fruits, eggs, fish and chicken (if you can't be vegetarian), and some sprouted whole grains.

"When I had colitis I could eat millet well cooked, whole grain rice and oatmeal, all of which provide B vitamins and fiber. I also could eat raw bananas, avocados, cantaloupes and honeydew mellons when I chewed them thoroughly. The only supplement I took was six grams a day of vitamin C in the form of sodium ascorbate powder. In just three weeks I was over the colitis. Dr. Silver was amazed.

"Last spring a combination of emotional shock, a fractured vertebrae and eating popcorn brought on colitis again. I immediately went on my colitis diet—with two changes. Each day I drank an eight ounce glass of juice extracted from leafy greens, including cabbage, leaf lettuce, spinach, beet tops, turnip tops, swiss chard, kale, comfrey and dandelion. At first I made it in the blender from a pint of packed leaves and six ounces of water and strained it. Then I got a juicer and took six ounces of pure juice. Instead of six grams of sodium ascorbate vitamin C, I took ten grams a day. In less than two weeks, no colitis."

"That's hard to believe."

"It is indeed. Don't take my word for it. Try it for yourself. Your weight will go down and so will your blood pressure while your energy and your spirits will soar."

Matilda's large, weary, protruding eyes looked at me with a kind of dark fire. "It's worth a try. Yes, it's worth a try."

"What have you got for us tonight, Elizabeth?" Nadine wanted to know as I came through the club house door for our next class session.

I set a basket down on the table. "Two surprises. One is a nutrition sheet for each of you whose problems we have touched upon thus far, with a list of personal aids for hygiene, skin care, reducing and general well being." I said, handing out the sheets.

"And the other surprise?" asked Janie.

"It's treats for all. Shall we have them now or at our break?"

"Now," everyone said. There was a childlike pleasure on their faces.

"We've agreed we don't need a break. We're all so interested we don't want to be interrupted," Ann said. She began setting out cups.

I poured hibiscus and elderberry tea and passed around the surprise, sugarless "candies" made of fruits, seeds and nuts.

Conversation was brisk with comments from everyone.

Betty set the pace right off with an exclamation of joy. "Look! I can raise my hands above my head. Two weeks of eating no sugar, no muscle meat, no processed foods and my arthritis pain is gone!" She held her arms above her head, smiling in triumph. "Oh yes, no citrus fruits."

"Betty, you said 'my' arthritis. Didn't we decide not to claim illness any more?" Sylvia said.

"We certainly did. God wants us to claim health," Flo said.

"Right," everybody echoed.

The group talked of the twenty-four-hour fast they had gone on, followed by the Dr. Coca pulse test for food allergies.

"A few foods made my heart accelerate about ten beats a minute," said Hilda who as yet had not discussed her problems. "But peanut butter—and it had no preservative in it—sent my heart to 100 beats a minute in twenty minutes and 120 beats at the end of an hour. I had a terrible headache. I was so exhausted and cross by bedtime, about two hours after I ate it, that I didn't care whether I lived or died."

Two of the girls reported their nighttime muscle cramps had stopped and Janie's cramps and muscle spasms were so noticeably better she radiated enthusiasm.

In ten minutes most of the tea cups were empty. Visiting quickly subsided.

"Andrea, would you like to be next?" I asked, turning to our youngest class member, an auburn-haired twenty-year-old. Although her weight had gone over normal for her by twenty pounds, her most serious problem was eyes. Her prospects for continued vision, according to her ophthalmologist, were not good. A few days before enrolling in the class she had told me about her ophthalmologist's report.

"I wear contact lenses for myopia," she had said. "The doctor discovered a tiny hole in the macula of my eyes."

"That's rather rare, isn't it?" I asked. I had just read of a famous biochemist having the same condition with that portion inside the eye where the image, coming through the lenses, focuses. He had saved his vision by maximum nutrition and some supplements.

"It's occasionally found in older people," Andrea had explained. "But I guess I'm the only young person to have the condition. At least the doctor has never heard or read of it."

She had told me she lived with a headache and nausea, that an allergist had found some of her food allergies but had attributed the headache and nausea to the eye condition. Andrea had quit seeing the allergist for several reasons. She could not afford the physician's high fees, she could not agree with him that much of her problem was psychological (she had basically a happy nature), nor that nutrition had little to do with the state of her health.

"You told me, Andrea, that you had gone to someone who advised you to have a hair analysis for minerals."

"Yes. Dr. Bonaman. I have a copy of the results for you." She handed me a folded sheet of paper. "Read it aloud if you like."

Because Elton had worked a great deal with nuclear spectroscopy and hair analysis was one of the many applied uses of that highly specialized field, we had become interested in the test. In the several years since, we had seen the results of many hair analyses.

When I glanced over Andrea's report, I got a real shock. Never had I seen such mineral deficiencies. These are the minerals that were drastically low: calcium, magnesium, sodium, potassium, zinc, phosphorus and iron. Her doctor told her the serum test results fairly well coincided with the hair analysis results.

No wonder Andrea could scarcely function well enough to hold down her bank job! She had been accepting her lack of health as psychological because of the many problems her parents and siblings had been going through. Only when the ophthamologist gave his verdict of her eye condition, had she been spurred on to do something about her health.

"Dr. Bonaman seemed puzzled by my hair analysis report," Andrea said after I had read it to the class.

"Did he give you some idea of what to do?"

"He gave me a prescription for potassium chloride tablets and told me to eat salty foods."

I bit my lips to keep quiet. When Dr. Silver noted on my first analysis that my serum sodium (salt) was eighty parts per million below the normal range (Andrea's was much lower) he had immediately prescribed a quarter teaspoon of salt in a glass of water after each meal, then told me to eat salty foods and to shake a little salt in drinking water between meals. In addition to the salt, he had me take supplements for the rest of the mineral deficiencies. Along with a balanced diet of high-vitamin foods, it took six months to bring my serum (blood) level of sodium up to low normal.

"Andrea, do you know what your blood pressure is?"

"Yes. My mother insisted it was a patient's right to know. It was 94/60."

"Do you have good energy?"

"I don't have good anything, much," she said with a slight giggle. Her soft voice belied her stark words.

"No wonder you don't have good energy. You need to get your blood pressure a little higher. I started with taking extra salt. A low blood pressure person oftentimes loses salt in the urine. You can test by putting a drop of urine on the end of your tongue. Urine's pure unless you've a bladder or kidney infection. Are you taking any medication?"

"Only a pain pill when my headache gets too bad for me to work."

"How often is that?"

"Nearly every afternoon."

"Anything else?"

"Not really. Unless you consider taking motion sickness pills. I get car sick when I go any distance. Our family doctor prescribed them when I was eight years old. He had my mother keep a bottle of tablets in the car. She gave me one whenever we went any place. I still take them when I ride for five miles or so."

I looked down to hide my distress. The pain pills she'd told me about were known to cause visual disturbances, digestive problems, nerve and heart malfunction and especially vitamins A and C deficiencies. That was bad enough. But the motion sickness pills were known to destroy vitamins, especially the B vitamins. Taken by Andrea since childhood, they may have contributed much to her appalling deficiencies and health problems.

"I'd like to go to Dr. Silver. Do you suppose he would see me?" Andrea asked.

"I'm sure he would," I replied, but he's very busy. People come to him from all over. You may have to wait for an appointment." I was vastly relieved to hear her request. Her many problems were so overwhelming they needed the attention of the best nutritionist-physician possible. Dr. Silver, I felt, was that person.

"In the meantime, could you give me some suggestions?": Her delft-blue eyes looked up, full of soul—eyes that could lose their sight within a year or so, plunging this lovely girl into darkness for the rest of her life.

"Of course. I may sound like a stuck record, but I cannot overemphasize what I'm about to repeat: eat *no* processed foods. None. In the grocery store go only to the fresh fruits and vegetables department; the dry legumes shelves for split peas, lentils, black-eyed peas, garbanzos and beans; the refrigerator section counter for eggs, the meat department for fresh or frozen fish. The health food store for refrigerated whole grain flours and cold-pressed salad oil with no chemical additives. Buy a sprouting book. You need the super nutrition of sprouted cereal grains, seeds, and legumes. And soak nuts in water for tastiness and ease of digesting.

"I'm allergic to many of those things."

"But not as allergic as you are to junk foods and processed foods with all the chemicals. If you can arrange for garden vegetables grown without commercial fertilizers and pesticides, by all means do so. I will test you kinesiologically for food allergies."

"There are some nuts and seeds I can eat."

"Wonderful. Buy only refrigerated ones. That is a must. All such things grow rancid, some very quickly, when out of refrigeration."

"What about vitamins?"

"You'll probably be allergic to something in the binders, to synthetics, to the vitamin source, as wheat for vitamin E, or lecithin made from soy and some of the B vitamins from yeast. You probably can take sodium ascorbate (vitamin C) in powder every day. I suggest two grams with each meal and two at bedtime. You may think that's a lot. But just remember that guinea pigs, a rare bat, primates and humans, through a fault in nature (mutation) don't synthesize vitamin C. But if humans did, they would synthesize between eight and fifteen grams a day, depending on size. If they had bacterial or viral infection, their body would synthesize between fifteen and thirty grams a day, just as goats, mice, elephants, snakes etc. do.

"Hopefully, you will get at least 1,000 milligrams (one gram) of vitamin C from those fresh foods you're going to be eating, mostly raw."

"What about the B vitamins? And vitamin A?"

"You told me you were allergic to brewer's yeast. Spirulina plankton also is excellent. Few people are allergic to it. It can also be bought under the name of chlorella, now produced in Japan. Many allergic people have found they can take that. Besides spirulina plankton (one half to one teaspoon or two to five tablets with meals), eat two cups of some leafy green vegetable each day, raw if you can. Or steamed or cooked two to three minutes in a little water. And drink the water.

"Before eating or cooking fresh vegetables and fruits bought at the supermarket, wash them in lukewarm water with suds made from ivory, castile, or handmade, unscented soap. That means *all* fresh foods. Even green leafy vegetables like lettuce, spinach, cabbage, kale. And strawberries and grapes. Many fruits and vegetables are not only sprayed during growth, they are sprayed with a chemical preservative at or near the time they leave the field so they will keep better during shipping and display in the grocery stores. Even fruits and vegetables you are going to peel should first be thoroughly washed and rinsed.

"Organically produced fresh foods need not be washed in soap suds unless they grow near a road or street where they have been frequently subjected to car exhaust fumes."

"Oh dear," Andrea sighed. "There's so much to learn. So many things that have to be done differently."

"If we are to survive," Sylvia said.

A moment of silence followed the statement. Everyone was

feeling the burden of responsibility for planning a nutritionally adequate diet for the stabilization of weight and the regaining of health.

The thought of the precious young girl, Andrea, possibly losing her sight from grave deficiencies rather overwhelmed me. I was glad it was time to dismiss the group.

When we met for another two hour session, Doris spoke up immediately. She was a small woman well past middle age with platinum hair and blue eyes that smiled. "I've had an operation for detached retina which took a long time to get over. Now my ophthalmologist says I have early-stage cataracts. And I still have high tension in my eyes—glaucoma—and bad water retention. He insists I take the maximum dosage of Thiuretic, a diuretic. I'm tired all the time and lately my knees and legs are weak and painful. And my balance is uncertain. That's all come about since taking the diuretic. I know it's that but the eye specialist says I don't dare leave off the medication."

"How effective is it?" I could see puffs under her eyes but her hands appeared slender.

"Oh, the pills work. He had me taking a tablet three times a day. But they made me feel light-headed and dizzy. I cut the dose to half a tablet three times a day and the feeling left, but the other symptoms are appearing."

"Was water retention noticeable before taking the diuretic?"

"Yes, I couldn't wear any rings. My watch band cut into my wrist and my ankles and feet looked like I had elephantitis. Could you tell us again which foods act as a diuretic?"

"First, let me ask you a question. Do you have a heart disorder?"

"No."

"Then your edema could be from kidney trouble or allergies. Is your blood pressure normal, high or low?"

"High."

"My husband got over edema, high blood pressure and glaucoma with a natural food diet." I told them he ate no sugar, dairy products, coffee or tea, muscle meat or animal fat and took megadoses of vitamin C. He followed the experience of Dr. Virno of the eye clinic, University of Rome, Italy. (Reported by Dr. Fred R. Klenner in his medical bulletin, "Observations on the Dose and Administration of Ascorbic Acid When Employed Beyond the Range of a Vitamin in Human Pathology.") Dr.

Virno gave five hundred milligrams of vitamin C per kilogram of body weight to glaucoma patients, with good results. Since my husband weighed about seventy-seven kilos, (170 pounds) the amount meant about thirty-eight grams of ascorbic acid which he took in two or three gram doses around the clock. In a six month period the pressure in his eyes went from twenty-six to fifteen, his blood pressure dropped to a high normal range, cholesterol changed from 290 to 140 and edema disappeared.

"Since then we've known of several people with one or all of those symptoms who have found very definite improvement following such a regimen. The best form of vitamin C to take in megadoses may be ascorbic acid powder, sold by health food stores and mail order vitamin companies. However, Dr. Linus Pauling, author of *Vitamin C and the Common Cold*, takes sodium ascorbate. The sodium does not act as sodium chloride (table salt) in the system.

"I'll do just what your husband did." "I almost forgot your question about diuretic foods, Doris. First I must report that ascorbic acid eight to fifteen grams a day, is a great diuretic. Foods that are diuretic are cucumber, watermelon, pineapple and asparagus, but all young green vegetables, rich in silicon, are excellent: alfalfa sprouts, any kind of leafy green vegetables, beets and their tops, garlic, onion, cabbage, parsnips. Apples, strawberries and grapes are good, as are cantaloupe and papayas. Nutritionist doctors say eat no meats, very little fish or eggs for awhile, and no dairy products unless you can't live that way. In that case take only small amounts of cottage cheese and yogurt or the soured milks.

"Moderate amounts of seeds—sesame, flax, sunflower and pumpkin—and some cereal grains as steel-cut oats, brown rice and millet. Better yet, sprouted cereal grains and buckwheat.

"When you eat watermelon, make a meal of it. Wash the rind with a nonchemical soap, rinse well and eat a three-by-four inch piece or juice all the rind. Mix the seeds with pieces of melon in a blender or juicer and strain. It makes excellent seed milk. In watermelon season, I eat a third of a ten pound one every day or so for breakfast—seeds, meat and rind. I never feel better or have more energy than when I eat such a breakfast. Whatever water retention I may have had (some air pollutants do that to me) leaves in hours."

"Oh, thank you Elizabeth. I'll go home and do all you suggested. I've got it written down." She held up her notebook, her small face aglow with purpose.

Connie's large, dark eyes were burning with anticipation. "You've already answered a lot of my questions. But a couple haven't been discussed. Maybe they're harder on my vanity than my health. I'm referring to the forty-seven extra pounds I can't get rid of and this change in skin pigmentation on my face, neck and arms." She lifted her chin so we could see her neck where the worst of the great splotches of white, pigmentless skin extended.

"And look at my arms." She pushed up her sleeves to show us more white patches.

We could all understand why she mentioned her suffering vanity, although she was anything but vain. In her late sixties, Connie continued to be a beautiful woman with high cheekbones, a sweet smile of near perfect teeth and platinum hair that framed her face in softly upswept curls. Her alternately pale olive and dead white skin was still fine textured and almost wrinkle-free.

"Your weight problem can be resolved with the diet program I will give you by the end of our course. And the vitiligo that would be most difficult for any of us to live with can be cleared up after your diet is unusually high in the natural source B vitamins."

"Are you implying my problem is malnutrition?"

I hadn't expected so blunt a question from tactful Connie. Since she said it with sweetness and humor, I answered directly. "Yes. Some cases have cleared up with daily doses of from 150 to 350 milligrams of pantothenic acid. Others have responded to 1,000 milligrams a day, or more, of PABA. But the quickest and most complete and lasting recovery comes from foods replete with all the B vitamins, like liver. One patient of a physician friend cleared up vitiligo in less than two weeks by eating one fourth pound of raw liver a day blended with V-8 juice. But your diet, Connie, though acting a bit slower, will be more appetizing. And it will include extra vitamin C."

"Someone said there's an ointment that helps."

"There is one that reportedly helps—PABA cream—sold in health food stores. Gently massaged in the affected areas of the skin, it may contribute to recovery. Remember what dermatologists say. Rub it twenty times for maximum absorption."

"I'll do it. Give myself every possible chance of recovery. To think that I've always prided myself in being a very special, gourmet cook! I caused my own downfall."

"And you'll pick yourself right up, I can see."

Esther, a black-haired, statuesque woman of striking personality, tilted back her head, and in unsmiling intensity, announced, "So I'm next. All of you know my problems since I recently got out of the hospital where you either wrote letters or visited me. My weight doesn't particularly bother me as weight. I've had it all my adult life. But my doctor insists I lose twenty pounds and so far I haven't been able to, in spite of appetite depressant pills and a high protein diet."

I prayed for the right thing to say to Esther. Four weeks before this class she had been rushed to the hospital by ambulance when she finally went to her doctor to show him the spontaneous bruises all over her extremities and body, and her blackish purple lips, gums, and tongue.

For two years she had been taking first Coumadin then Dicumarol, anticoagulants for a blood and heart condition. During a visit to her doctor to report dizziness and weakness, he had given her a heart medicine with anticoagulant in it without decreasing the dosage of the pure anticoagulant. The extra anticoagulant in the heart medicine thinned her blood too much.

Esther was put in intensive care and given blood transfusions. When she came home from the hospital she looked haggard and pale. Only the last week or two had she begun to perk up.

She was another victim of over medication and under nutrition. While Esther was in the hospital, I consulted *The Physician's Desk Reference* to learn the side effects of Dicumarol that she was still taking. Like medical diuretics, it strongly tended to cause deficiencies of the B vitamins, magnesium, potassium and many other nutrients. Magnesium and potassium are essential for preventing heart attacks, the very happening the doctor was trying to avoid in Esther. Yet the more Dicumarol (or Coumadin) she took, the more she contributed to deficiencies that contributed to the heart problem.

"I will help you to lose weight. In the meantime, try very hard to quit coffee. You said you fell in love with hibiscus tea. I've a good supply. I'll see that you get some tomorrow."

Esther still lived on the brink of disaster. I determined to get her diet regimen ready for her and deliver it with the tea. My heart ached for her, another victim of a dangerous drug and vicious circle syndrome.

After a brief recess, I turned to Hilda and smiled. "Thank you for being so patient. It's rarely easy to be last."

"Last but not *least*," she quipped, dropping her hands and extending her arms at the elbows to emphasize her bulk. A sad, wistful smile lingered on her thin lips.

It was difficult to imagine that this forty-five-year-old, excessively obese woman shaking constantly with Parkinson's disease, had once been a strawberry-blond, Power's girl model. Disillusioned and cynical, Hilda was nevertheless sympathetic and sensitive to the troubles of others in spite of appearing to be withdrawn. Generous to a point of poverty for herself, this freelance writer existed mainly on canned soup, pastas and a few herbs from a tiny patio garden.

Hilda quickly went on. "Once about two years ago, I fasted for five days."

From her sad expression I could not discern whether the experience had been satisfactory or disastrous. "That's very interesting," I said, groping for the right words.

"We'd like to hear about it." Ann, ever the impulsive one, said.

The whole class added an enthusiastic yes.

"There's not all that much to tell. I had read Charles Bragg's book on fasting. I was broke—no money at all—and waiting for the check for an article assignment I'd completed. The first two days of the fast I felt so lousy I stayed in bed. The next two weren't much better except that I didn't shake. What a relief. The fifth day I felt good. Really great. Then the check came and I started eating."

"How did you break the fast?"

"With fruit juice. Then a salad. I wasn't too awfully hungry and felt satisfied with a glass of most any kind of juice, a salad or vegetable soup."

"Good for you! How long did you continue on this excellent program?"

Hilda gave a short, cynical laugh. "About three days. Then an old friend from New York arrived and insisted we celebrate my article being published. I thought, oh what the hell. So I got back to drinking. And eating all wrong. And shaking. God, how I shook. I couldn't write and suddenly I was nearly broke so I went to Alcoholics Anonymous.

"Well, I'm not drinking and I am writing some again. But I'm eating and shaking. The doctor I go to says I must reduce but hasn't suggested how. He says I should eat something of

everything but just half as much. He did have me take vitamin
B6 for awhile but it did no good. A lot of my weight is water
retention. When I take the Dyazide he gave me my weight goes
down ten or fifteen pounds, but I feel lousy again. I'm weak,
nauseated, dizzy, have a headache, muscle cramps and bruises all
over that I can't account for. And I can't write. My head's
nothing but a cork. So I stop the diuretic and—well, its a circle of
torment except for my weight which is torture. That goes up
and up. I'm over two hundred pounds in spite of a high protein
diet. Can you believe my normal weight should be a hundred and
ten?"

Hilda looked straight at me, her face distorted with anguish
and loneliness. She was a newcomer in our midst and to my
knowledge, had no local friends.

"And that will be your normal weight again, Hilda."

"You are the only one who thinks so." Tears glistened in her
eyes. "My doctor says I must learn to live with a fatty liver and
Parkinson"s disease. He tried nerve cytotrophin which I
thought helped some but it didn't last. And later he gave me L-
dopa. That helped too, but not for very long."

Hilda had indicated that she ate a high protein diet. I
wondered if her doctor had cautioned her sufficiently to eat very
little meat while taking the L-dopa. The Levadopa (generic
name), an amino acid forerunner of dopamine, has been found
to be effective in some clinical use and studies. But a high
protein diet upsets that effective action.

"The body has marvelous recuperative powers and reserves.
Your fast proved that. Once all the impurities, the toxic
substances are thrown off, the body functions beautifully, and
given the proper materials, can restore itself. Those materials
are the natural, untreated foods in the right amounts. They are
the building blocks. They can build back the damaged cells of the
organs. If thousands of us are experiencing recovery from grave
degenerative diseases, then you can too. However, it takes time
and patience and usually some setbacks beyond our control."

"Time is what I've got a lot of. I'll work on the patience. How
do I get started?"

"You've made a most remarkable start. You've quit alcohol
and you've proven that you can fast."

"What causes the Parkinson's disease? What deficiencies, I
suppose I should ask?"

"The experts say deficiencies of probably all the B vitamins with B6 at the top of the list. It takes a lot of repair nutrients. A car with 150,000 miles on it can't be overhauled with just a new battery. It needs a lot of new parts. Like a much used car, we all need more than just one repair part. You mentioned muscle cramps."

"Yes. I've had many. For years before Parkinson's disease set in. I've been taking a teaspoonful of milk of magnesia since you talked about it in class and I'm better. I can even walk a little straighter." She smiled with the sudden realization that already she had started to improve. "And I took a lot of notes on the diet for edema."

"Then you're on your way. I'll have a nutrition program worked up for you by the next class. In the meantime, one more thing. That list of foods will be planned to be eaten raw. It will be low in protein. Can you find raw goat's milk around here?"

"I don't know, but I can buy frozen goat's milk in Seattle." She laughed and made some feeble joke about being a kid at heart. But her face showed a mixture of sadness and discouragement overlaid with a wan expression of hope.

The class ended with the girls all laughing with her and giving her a prolonged handclap while generously voicing their encouragement.

As Hilda, trembling and uncertain, struggled to her feet and steadied herself to walk out to her car, I asked God to give her strength and courage, patience and trust sufficient for her great need.

An overweight person's downfall is often her appetite. I confess I used the lure of food the last session to impress my class.

"What fun to come here for our last meeting," Ann's voice sang out above the chatter of the others as they filed into our living room.

"And what a beautiful buffet," exclaimed Sylvia.

"Losing weight can be fun even though it requires hard work," I said.

"Did you prepare all that food yourself, Elizabeth?" Flo asked.

"No. I confess a friend helped me." Several of the foods required last minute preparation. I served green cocktail with dandelion juice, a sprinkling of celery seeds, a few drops of lemon juice and sesame oil, hot, raw pea soup, floating soup croutons made of sprouted (budded) garbanzos.

"I see an exotic bread," Nadine said.

"All-buckwheat. Made from an all-rye bread recipe."

"Is that real butter, Elizabeth?" Connie wanted to know.

"Yes, raw butter blended with an equal part of safflower oil. It makes soft, spreadable butter."

"I'll bet there's no dessert, Elizabeth," Betty teased.

"Maybe some wouldn't call it dessert. I'll let you be the judge. It's fresh fruits with cookies made of ground raisins and coconut."

With the food all ready, I served the class immediately. While we ate, we listened to tapes on hypoglycemia, on the importance of minerals in body metabolism, and on nutrition for weight loss stressing an ovo-lacto, mostly raw vegetarian fare. As they ended and we finished eating, I brought out my handiwork.

"Here are the nutritious programs I promised the rest of you. They provide 1,600 to 2,400 calories a day, depending first on activity, then on height and frame size. What is restricted are animal fats and proteins. The average American gets between fifty and sixty percent of calories from fats, mostly animal. I've suggested getting half that many calories from mostly vegetable fats. Butter, no more than one pat. *No* hydrogenated oils and margarines. They are all so highly processed and nutritionless no creature on earth but man will voluntarily eat them. With almost no nutrients in them there is nothing to spoil. They have a shelf life of forever.

"These nutrition plans include little or no muscle meat. Meat eating in the life of mainstream America provides way over the amount of protein the body needs for maintenance and repair. That extra protein has to be converted, by the liver, to calories. That conversion is hard labor for the liver. It uses so much body energy the person may be left too tired and sluggish for activity sufficient to burn up those calories. And so—they are stored as fat.

"Wow!" Ann's face brightened with smiles. "Now if I can just keep from cheating, I'll be ready for a bikini by the time I'm a grandmother."

"Elizabeth, I can't lose weight on a thousand calories a day, let alone 2,000."

"Remember the fat-burning hormone somatotropin and what to eat to produce it. Then think exercise." To myself I called Sylvia a "go" girl. She had a new small car, and because it used little gas, indulged her whims to go places. She rarely stayed home. I knew she neither hiked, gardened nor did home exercises.

"Join our yoga class, Sylvia," Dottie suggested.

"You meet on choir practice night," Sylvia's answer was defensive.

"Then jog with me along the beach every day at 6:30 a.m." Flo said.

"I didn't know you jogged," Sylvia exclaimed.

"I don't. But I'm going to. My husband's promised to take care of the baby if he wakes up before I get back."

The house was silent as a mountain top after the last friendly voice said goodbye. I sat alone before our fireplace, for Elton had gone to Seattle and wouldn't be back until late.

What had I accomplished with the class, I asked myself. Perhaps a start on the long road to good health. Hopefully some sustaining encouragement, a will to follow the food regimen and enough curiosity to read the books I included in a short bibliography to help them to help themselves.

I wished I had stressed the importance, the necessity, of each adult working out his or her own nutrition program, exercises, positive philosophy and faith.

Part IV

Our Personal Stories

Elizabeth Triumphs Over Cancer

My cancer story began, I have no doubt, in 1952, when I was given the maximum dosage of the "miracle" antibiotic, Chloromycetin, for pneumonia. It truly changed my life. I recovered in record time, but I continued to run a low grade temperature for a year and a half. From then on I was very susceptible to colds and flu and ran a fever for months after recovering. My energy level was so low I was unable to do any physical work or even walk a block. Between such periods, which represented about half the time, I had only fair energy and little endurance.

Not until some ten years after taking the Chloromycetin did I learn that it could, and in most cases did, destroy bone marrow where the white blood (defense) cells are made! This knowledge at least answered the nagging question as to why my white count in every blood test showed twenty per cent of normal.

From the time of the Chloromycetin episode, my health began to go down. In 1977 cancer was diagnosed. I experienced so many different health problems it's hard to conceive of them all. Eighteen of those twenty-five years I went from one doctor to another, to many clinics and laboratories for special tests, landed in several hospitals for surgery I didn't need and special treatments that proved useless or harmful. In 1970 when my husband, a chemist, realized that certain prescription drugs I was taking were the cause of near fatal potassium deficiency, he began to encourage and help me to take my health care into my own hands. "I'll help you in every way I can. You have the determination, the persistence it takes," he said.

Deep into nutrition study from then on, I struggled for survival day by day, week by week, year by year. I fought "terminal" Addison"s disease (the doctor gave me no more than two years to live), arthritis, colitis, duodenal ulcer, alternate diarrhea and constipation, severe ecological allergies, tic douloureux, hiatus hernia, shingles, osteoporosis, chronic indigestion, bursitis and bronchitis, to mention a partial list of diseases that wracked my body. Gradually I conquered most of them, including hemorrhoids and the painful, bleeding intestinal polyps I had almost consented to have removed by surgery. Despite freedom from many of these ills the conventional medical profession considers incurable or untreatable without surgery and drugs, I still had to reckon with anemia.

Then when I passed black, coagulated blood clots, I feared something ominous was happening. Because I'd been for several years on a natural, fifty percent raw diet, with all allergy-causing foods eliminated, I felt I would never have cancer. I was wrong. After learning I had a malignant tumor in the ascending colon (a dull pain had plagued me for two years), I realized it had been present a long time. As it was a slow growing kind, my nutritionist physician said it had probably started between fifteen or twenty years before, maybe even longer. I also had had for years small skin cancers on my face and a large one on the back of my hand.

With the positive verdict of cancer of the ascending colon, the doctors immediately set plans in motion for taking care of the cancer. The procedure was routine. My case, according to them, was just another of the type they dealt with every day. The surgery they began to discuss would probably result in a colostomy. Then there would be chemotherapy and radiation. How many months or years it would continue could only be determined as I "progressed."

I was shocked at how established, how automated, how categorized, how narrow was the path of this drastic, destroying treatment. I would almost be like a thing on the conveyor belt of an assembly line. Yet I was an individual. Different. Unique. No two people are ever alike in any way for a multitude of reasons. I had already learned there were many alternate therapies for diseases. I had already proven to myself with God's constant guidance, with Elton's optimism, encouragement and help, and my own efforts, my body could conquer them. God gave us a marvelous creation in the form of our body. It was made to self-heal if treated the way He intended. I thought of the Bible that teaches us how to nourish ourselves the way He originally intended. "I give every seed-bearing plant on the face of the whole earth and every tree that has fruit with seed in it. They will be yours for food." Gen: 1–29, and "...the tree of life bearing twelve crops of fruit, yielding its fruit every month— and leaves—for the healing of the nations." Rev: 22–2.

Politely, quietly, I listened to the plans for the dreadful, drastic ordeal the doctors laid out for me. I left without saying a word, not because I was overwhelmed for my own welfare, but because I saw an otherwise slow death running full speed in the hands of determined physicians whose minds were closed to the wishes of the patient. The natural, painless constructive ways of healing God taught us to employ were beyond their comprehension.

In the fresh air outside the hospital clinic, I made my decision. God was looking down on me with great understanding. He stood by me in love and compassion. His words rang like clear bells in my mind. "I will never leave thee." And the indwelling of the Holy Spirit filled me with peace and the assurance of recovery. I was joyous. I was radiant. I knew the direction I would *not* take: the direction that led to the "cut, poison and burn" modalities of surgery, drugs and radiation.

Years of nutrition study had prepared me for this decision. Elton's loving support would help me stay with it. I recalled reading the booklet of Christine Nolfi, M.D., of Denmark. She cured herself of breast cancer by an all-raw diet. If she could, I could, I told myself. I also had read Ann Wigmore's *Be Your Own Doctor*, which bolstered my confidence.

At that time Elton was away for two weeks. I had decided to stay home, consult the internist about the pain in my side, then do some shopping for our October trip to Australia and New Zealand with the International College of Applied Nutrition.

When I met my returning dear one at the airport, we were so caught up in happiness on seeing each other and chatting about his successful trip, I could not bring myself to tell him about the verdict of cancer. As the hours spun by in joy and sharing, I decided *not* to tell him. There was no reason to. Although my health was not vigorous, it was good enough to withstand the mild rigors of today's travel. Besides, he might have cancelled our reservations in an effort to protect me, had he known. That would have been a tremendous disappointment to him.

By touring Australia and New Zealand in their spring, we would find an abundance of fresh fruit and vegetables for my raw diet. We did, and I enjoyed the trip immensely, benefiting from it in many ways.

Why a raw diet? Because from thirty to eighty-five percent of the nutrition in natural foods is destroyed in cooking. That is an average of fifty percent loss! I knew a cancer patient could not afford to eat anything that is not health giving if he or she wanted to get well.

There are two more reasons for eating raw foods. Cancer cells proliferate only where there is not enough oxygen for cells to be healthy. Give the area and the whole body optimal oxygen and the cancer can't proliferate. *Raw foods contain an abundance of oxygen. In cooked foods oxygen is destroyed.* This is a powerful fact. A truth. Jesus said, "Ye shall know the truth and the truth shall make ye free." I *knew* some day I would be free of cancer if I learned to use the patience and persistence God gave me.

The other reason for eating only living (raw) foods is they give more energy. They contain *all* nutrients for energy intact, unaltered. They digest so easily only ten percent of one's total energy is used. Conventional, mostly cooked and processed foods take thirty percent of total energy for digestion. It means anyone on an all raw diet has at least twenty percent more energy than the average person. Actually, figuring other factors such as far fewer toxins (processed foods are full of toxic additives that take their toll in energy expenditure by requiring they be thrown off) and reduced body function efficiency, we find even more than a twenty percent bonus in energy for the living foods person. It's more like fifty percent more energy for the raw food eater than the average eater.

For me there was every reason for an all raw diet and none against. Not one. What a joy it was! Besides, I much preferred the delicious, natural taste. The extra blessing was Elton's acceptance of uncooked menus. "Don't bother to fix me anything different, honey," he would say before we started preparing dinner. "I'll just eat what you eat."

My cancer battle was not the toughest one I ever fought but it was the longest—two years and two months. My first great skirmish was discovering I had to eat more than just the fruits and vegetables, and the few seeds and nuts the ten or twelve raw food books advocated. Hunger, the powerful motivator, spurred me on to learn of all the raw foods available, how to sprout every kind of edible seed, then figure out ways I could prepare them to satisfy my taste, cravings and weight needs.

It didn't take long to do that. But writing it in a form acceptable for publication that would answer the myriad questions audiences, classes and counselees asked, took nearly a year. That publication, *The UNcook Book,* is, in essence, the account of the way I conquered cancer: the foods, the supplements, the green drinks containing dandelion and comfrey, and the wheat grass juice. The how-to's. The don'ts. The whys. It does not say anything about exercises which was a daily part of my recovery program. That is in *Bandwagon To Health,* the book that followed. But neither tells the final chapter of my cancer battle story, a skirmish that nearly ended in tragedy, the tragedy of failure, of surgery, of chemotherapy and of radiation.

It was early March, 1979, and we were returning from Mexico on planes that missed connections. We endured trying unexpected situations, fatigue and finally unusually raw cold weather upon returning to our home on Puget Sound. My low immune system could not cope with the severe bronchial pneumonia I sank into. With intravenous vitamin C for a week in a hospital, I was up again, but barely so. The usual low grade temperature following a respiratory infection kept me so throttled I was more down than up. In May, realizing I was not progressing, I went for three weeks to a living foods health resort I had been to before. I left after two weeks to go home to bed. I was ill. Summer passed quickly because I was writing *The UNcook Book* all the time in bed.

But by mid August I realized I needed help. Because of a real obstruction in the lower right side of my colon, my digestive system was hardly functioning. As I was suffering a peculiar allergy, I went to see my internationally known allergist. She took one look at me and demanded, "Have you got cancer? You are ashy white." I think she wanted to scare me into action. I told her of the diagnosis two years before and my other baffling problems. She interrupted me to take the bandage off my hand. "That's a skin cancer," she said, giving the dime size lesion a long scary name. "That's a deep one. How long has it been there?" I told her seven years. "Have it removed before it involves the tendons any more," she scolded. I smiled but thought a frown. Surgery might remove it but it would mutilate my hand, leave vast scar tissue and probably permanently cripple my fingers. I had seen such a surgery-riddled hand.

The good lady continued. "I want you to go to University Hospital and get a Carcenoembryonic Antigen Test (CEA) tomorrow." She wrote out the order as soon as she finished taking care of my allergy and dismissed me with a short, "I'll call you."

A week to the day she called me. "You're as high as you can be on the positive side of the CEA test," she declared. I felt sure she was trying to push me to what she felt was the logical, the safe, sane, physical, visual approach to handling cancer. Conventional doctors have to "see" their cases by X-ray, laser, fluoroscope, special lights or an incision that lays open the innards. They seem to find it increasingly difficult to "believe" the invisible healing God has for us for the asking. It is His gift. I asked her what she would suggest I do. Her answer was quick and sure. "Find the best possible colon cancer surgeon and have that tumor out immediately." I asked another question or two to avoid any comment, thanked her and hung up.

"Oh Lord, my precious Lord," I prayed," you'll have to tell me again what to do. Do you really not want me to have surgery? I'm all out of ideas. I've come to the end of my resources. Shall I have surgery?" Elton took me in his arms. "It's all right, honey. Just hang in there. God has a way. He'll let you know," he said. I could feel the warm blanket of his love wrap around me. As we drove home, his words of assurance repeated over and over in my mind.

It was about 10:30 A.M., and I lay exhausted. In limbo physically, spiritually, mentally. Weakness and the sharp pains of indigestion enveloped me. Had I missed God's will for me? Was I at the end of my narrow road full of rocks, chuckholes, ominous overhanging cliffs? Was I not going to make it through the valley of the shadow of death? I prayed fervently, but went to sleep before I finished. When I awoke at 1:00 P.M., Elton was standing over me with a little dish of fresh peaches he'd pureed in the blender. When he learned I did not dare add more food to my small undigested breakfast, his face fell. "Honey, I've been thinking. Maybe you'd better water fast. What do you think?" We discussed it briefly before I agreed. I dreaded the long, lonely sleeplessness a fast meant for me.

That was Friday morning, the beginning of my fast. The following Tuesday morning I awoke feeling better, but so weak Elton had to help me to the bathroom. We had been in touch each day with the doctor on the Oregon coast who, six years before, had supervised my seven-day diagnostic fast that left me well and wise to the allergy-causing foods that had been making me so very ill up to that time. When Elton reported to him the morning situation, he agreed with our suggestion to continue with a juice fast.

We started with two ounces of fresh-made apple juice diluted with water, and continued with a different kind and increased amount of freshly extracted juice every three hours. My digestion was functioning. I felt better and progressively had more energy. The morning of the eighth day of the water-juice fast I went to the bathroom for a wonderful elimination. It was huge, of proper consistency, diameter and color. With it came a large greenish-blackish, firm dense mass about three and one half inches long, two inches wide and three quarters of an inch thick. Somehow I knew beyond a shadow of a doubt it was the old dead tumor. I yelled for Elton to come. On seeing it he was as excited as I. We laughed and cried and hugged and kissed. From that day on, my health improved steadily. I felt so cleansed, so clear-headed, so near to my Maker. The low grade fever I had had since the March pneumonia, faded away. I began to gain in energy and weight. By December I felt well. I had finished *The Uncook Book,* sent it off to the publisher and we were preparing for lecturing in California enroute to our winter home in Mexico. I felt great but I had to *know* what the doctors wouldn't believe because they could not *see* any proof. Again I took the CEA test. Afterwards we drove on to California. Soon after we arrived, our number two son in Portland called to give us the report of the CEA test. All clear. No cancer. That was wonderful news. To be doubly sure, we consulted several alternate cancer specialists. Two had had patients who passed their cancerous tumors when the walls of the colon healed and expelled the intruding cancer. A colonic specialist we talked to said she'd had three patients pass their cancers when the colon became healthy. She explained the difference between a dead, undissolved, little-shrunken tumor and a rubberlike mass of old, colon mucus. The tumor has threadlike, black, wiggly lines all through it. They are the dead blood of the fine veins of the tumor, she explained.

Again, we were assured but felt there was one last step in putting to rest the story of my cancer. I had the Dr. Harold Harper test and the Arthur-Amid test. Both showed no sign of cancer. There was still another assurance, an unplanned one. Just before leaving San Diego for Mexico, I took off the adhesive bandage, showered and started to gently dry my hand as I'd had to do for seven years. But there was no need to be careful. The cancer was gone. No more deep, flaking scab the size of a dime. Only wonderful, smooth, clean skin with such a tiny scar I could scarcely see it—just enough to keep me reminded and thankful. How beautiful is healing! How great are God and Jesus and the Holy Spirit who saw me through the valley of the shadow of death.

Elton Masters Glaucoma

In 1967, Elizabeth and I were sued by a former employee whom we had put through accounting school and later made our assistant manager. We were accused of collusion. Even though we were eventually completely exonerated, the sustained trauma of that experience did great damage to our health, peace of mind and confidence.

The most serious problem resulting from that ordeal subtly crept up on me a year and a half later. I had glaucoma. "The tension in your eyes is very high," the opthalmologist said after the examination. "We'll have to operate. We don't want to risk detached retina." I paused a moment then told him I would think it over, thanked him and left for home.

I had recalled Elizabeth telling me about high doses of vitamin C for the relief and recovery of glaucoma. When I got home, she went to our files and took out a booklet by Frederick R. Klenner. It was full of medical information and case histories of patients he had successfully treated with megadoses of vitamin C. In the booklet he told about two ophthalmologists at the University of Rome who were effectively treating glaucoma with vitamin C. Their patients were greatly improved or recovered. The amount of vitamin C to be taken was sensibly arrived at, I thought, by a simple formula: 500 milligrams of vitamin C powder (fine crystals) per kilogram of normal body weight per day. My 170 pounds translated to seventy-seven kilos, which meant thirty-eight grams of vitamin C to be taken each day, distributed in doses around the clock.

As chairman of the Physics Department and teaching both physics and a class in physical chemistry, I worked a long day. Every morning, first thing, Elizabeth measured thirty-eight grams of ascorbic acid fine crystals, another name for vitamin C, in a small bottle for me to carry. I took two grams (one half teaspoon) about every hour through the day and evening; and three grams before bed. When the alarm went off at 2:00 A.M. I took four grams. The first thing I did on arising was to take the remaining ascorbic acid crystals. By the time I showered, dressed and had breakfast, it was time to start the next thirty-eight grams of vitamin C.

At first, it seemed to me all I got done was to dissolve vitamin C in water! I took it with a straw to keep it off my teeth, because ascorbic acid can gradually eat the enamel of the teeth and turn them brown. But in a week or so the chore became so routine I was able to pretty well forget it and carry on with life as usual.

After a few days of studying up on the efficacy of vitamin C in all sorts of body functions, including the eyes, Elizabeth and I decided I didn't need to take the eye drops that were supposed to relieve the tension and ache there. I never did use the artificial tears. In a couple of weeks my eyes felt fine. Only occasionally after an especially long, involved day, did I have eye ache or burning in my eyes. After awhile that ceased altogether.

At that time, 1968, Elizabeth was just beginning to get into improved nutrition. We cut down on sugar, canned foods, prepared, pre-cooked foods, cured and lunch meats. We still had red meat four or five times a week but we did change to brown rice, whole wheat flour and products, and more fresh vegetables and fruits.

After seven months of taking thirty-eight grams of vitamin C every day, and feeling fine, I went to see the opthalmologist. He examined my eyes without saying a word. He led me to another examining cubicle and examined them again. Looking puzzled, he excused himself, left and soon brought back two colleagues. They both examined my eyes with their instruments. Finally they all mumbled a few words together in apparent agreement and my doctor spoke. "For some reason, you do not have glaucoma." He hesitated and I studied his puzzled face, wondering what his problem was. Then incredibly he said, "But we should go ahead and operate." I told him I wanted to go home and think it over. Thanking him and the other two doctors, I left.

I never went back. Elizabeth did later. She got a copy of all my records before and after the vitamin C therapy.

The amazing thing to me is that vitamin C worked its miracle without the ideal accompaniment of optimal diet, and in a body that had asthma, high blood pressure, high cholesterol, varicose veins, a chemically damaged liver and poorly functioning intestines. Let me say, however, that there was *improvement* in all those problems as well. A few years later, I went on Elizabeth's all-natural, vegetarian diet of living foods and overcame those problems almost entirely.

There's a sequel to the glaucoma story. Through the years since that miraculous time, my eyes have continued to improve, as evidenced by less strong lenses every three or four years. Each time the doctor comments on the healthy tissue in my eyes. I thank God for leading us to the natural therapies that help our bodies to heal themselves. Vitamin C is needed in abundance by the eyes. It's one of the organs that needs to store some vitamin C because stress is immediately reflected in the eyes, subtly or noticeably, and vitamin C helps protect us from harmful effects of stress. A few years after this experience scientists learned there's a vitamin C complex—hesperidin, rutin and several other substances found in the pulp of fruits, especially the white of the skin of citrus fruits. That complex is called bioflavonoids. It makes vitamins much more efficiently metabolized by the body.

Part V

Appendix

Why A Vegetarian Diet

The case for a vegetarian diet has been covered in the text of this book. Here we will review some of the main reasons for such a way of life.

As far as we're concerned there is no case against a vegetarian diet. However, nonvegetarians disagree. Their main reason is powerful. Correctly they point out that vitamin B12, the antianemia factor, is essential for normal blood. Since vitamin B12 is found only in animal products (meat, fowl, fish and eggs), it must be eaten for that vital nutrient. Right?

Wrong. A few years ago, research and studies revealed vitamin B12 is in many deep root plants such as alfalfa, winter wheat, winter squash, dandelion, nopal cactus (a close relative of prickly pear that grows over most of the lower half of the United State), comfrey, aloe vera, and edible dock, to mention a few. And the single, most abundant source of vitamin B12 is a plant, spirulina plankton and blue-green algae. *It is twice as replete with vitamin B12 as the most abundant animal source, liver!*

Recent bioscientists have turned up this fact: the healthy intestine synthesizes vitamin B12 from ingested natural foods. If we are truly healthy, as vegetarians are apt to be, we need not struggle to find those less usual plants and have them consistently in our diet. We can relax and enjoy while our intestines manufacture sufficient vitamin B12 from unprocessed carbohydrates to keep us healthy.

Another point nonvegetarians invariably bring up is the matter of protein. They are often downright scared they will waste away, lose what health they have, enjoy little energy and grow old fast without the assured proteins of flesh eating.

Actually, quite the opposite is true. Since adults and growing children need between twenty-five and forty-five grams of protein a day instead of the fifty-five to 125 grams a day medical science advocated from the mid nineteenth century until the 1960's, it is easy to understand how a vegetarian diet of good variety can measure up to the protein requirement.

There is protein in all plants, more of course in their seeds, which we should also eat. Meat eaters tend to eat too much protein. What is not used by the body for maintenance and repair has to be converted to calories to be burnt up by activity or stored as fat in the body. This is one great reason why meat eaters are often overweight. The conversion of protein unused for maintenance and repair puts extra strain on the liver, which means it takes extra energy, leaving less energy for body activity. It is probably why, after eating meat, a person is apt to feel sluggish. Here are a few review points on living the vegetarian way:

1. Man has the teeth for biting off and chewing, and the lengthy intestines for digesting crisp, hard, fibrous foods.

2. He doesn't have the extremely acid stomach of carnivores for properly breaking down ingested animal protein. As a result, meats stay in the intestines forty-eight to 100 hours, becoming putrefactive and toxic, a poison that is reabsorbed into the bloodstream, making that stream very impure.

3. A vegetarian diet rarely puts excess fat on the body.

4. Meat eating is the most expensive way to get protein into our bodies. Why put all those wonderful high protein plants and seeds through an animal to make him grow to prime size, pay for the expensive procedure of getting him to market, butchered, processed, put through the costly handling of the slaughter house, the wholesaler, and the retailer to get to your kitchen? You have to spend time and fuel to prepare it for the table, and more time to clean up the greasy mess it leaves on kitchen walls, dishes and utensils. Why not eat the delicious plants and seeds themselves, preferably raw, at a *lot less cost,* at no danger of making you fat while giving you more energy and a clearer mind?

5. Vegetarians live longer and are freer of disease. Seventh Day Adventists who are usually vegetarian, drink no

coffee, tea or alcohol, live the longest. Mormans who consume little meat, coffee, tea or alcohol are close behind. Both groups have less degenerative disease than other population groups.

6. People who have overcome cancer the natural way have usually eliminated flesh entirely from the diet.

7. Athletes, such as long distance runners, find they have more endurance when they eat all vegetarian fare, mostly raw. Our nephew who went through college on scholarships earned by his performance in distance running, found this to be especially true.

A young Australian friend, a member of the Natural Health Society of Australia, Canberra Chapter, told us he had less energy the morning after eating meat. Cooked starch, such as rice, baked potato, pasta or white flour bread, also lessened his morning gusto. It was difficult to believe one cooked starch would make a noticeable difference in a person's reserve energy. So Elizabeth had to experiment for herself.

She chose a medium size yam, a starch that agreed with her, either cooked or raw. Three different times, several days apart, she felt good and was not under extra stress. She ate the raw yam with the same raw menu, enjoying a quiet evening at home, and sleeping her required six to six and one half hours. The morning after, she felt full of vigor and was able to indulge in her vigorous exercise program, of seventeen army push-ups.

Three different times, several days apart, feeling good and not under stress, she ate a cooked yam and the same raw menu for dinner. Although feeling good each morning after, she was not able to do the seventeen push-ups. Twelve was the limit one morning, and fourteen was the absolute limit the other two mornings. Since that time, when eating out and taking a helping of some cooked starch, she notices less energy for her vigorous exercises.

Remember: it takes thirty percent total energy to digest a conventional diet of mostly cooked, processed foods that include meat. It takes ten percent total energy to digest an uncooked diet, even less if mostly fruit and sprouts are eaten. You never feel sluggish. If you find this difficult to accept, try it for yourself. If you are healthy, you'll have twenty percent more energy and feel great.

Why shouldn't plant foods provide the way for the body to

maintain vigorous health, to prevent sickness, to heal itself? It is the natural way, the way God originally taught us.

The Advantages of Organically Grown Food

Organically grown, unsprayed vegetables, fruits, grains, nuts and seeds are the ideal foods. "Organically grown" is a general terminology applied to plants cultivated in soils fed with natural compost as opposed to chemical fertilizers. Inorganic growers say their crops are more abundant, just as rich in nutrition, and the only way that is economically feasible for them to continue in their farming business. Laboratory test claims are made by both sides of the organic/inorganic controversy, each claiming equal or superior quality of harvested crop.

It takes no gourmet or expert in flavors, however, to detect the superior taste of fresh produce grown in soils where the naturally occurring nutrients are put back into the soil each year. They are decidedly more delicious than the same food grown in the same area and climate but fertilized with from two to five kinds of chemical substances. One has only to garden organically to prove the difference. People who test weak on chemically fertilized produce from the supermarket usually test strong on produce organically grown. Methods that turn from the natural way are apt to lead us all astray.

Following organic gardening plus organic fruit and nut tree cultivation are all important if you have a bit of space. If you don't have space read our book, *Bandwagon to Health.* Even the tiniest kitchen can become a food-producing garden of superb nutritious edibles at a fraction of the cost of grocery store foods.

The Merits of Health Food Stores

Health food stores are so under attack at this writing, they are in danger of being closed. Propaganda against them comes from a variety of vested interests. Much of it is untrue, exaggerated and wholly unjust. Another freedom in our great country will be lost if legislators yield to pressure from highly financed entities and pass laws to close these small businesses.

Health food stores serve a real purpose. They sell rare and whole foods found in only a very few other outlets such as co-ops, specialty shops and ethnic food stores in large cities. Where but in your health food store would you find dry peas that sprout to become one of the most delicious, nutritious foods known? (Despite the price, they turn out to be cheaper than canned or frozen peas.) Or fresh, raw nuts of all kinds kept under *refrigeration* so they don't go rancid? Where else would you find whole grain, no-wheat bread (refrigerated) for the countless persons allergic to gluten? Or sun dried fruits that haven't been treated with poisonous sulfur dioxide to keep them moist? Even without all those vitamin, enzyme and mineral supplements that people wish to buy, there would still be good reasons for the modest little health food store to exist—to carry specialty foods so helpful to so many of us.

It is true, health food stores have some drawbacks. They are often more expensive because they can't buy in the huge quantities chain grocers can. And yes, there are some items which are processed or contain sugar or artificial sweeteners. If we read labels, however, we can avoid those products. Because they are there is no reason to close the store. We are not required to buy them. We can refuse them. But without health food stores and co-ops many Americans would be hard pressed to find the items they need to eat healthily.

High, Medium and Low Energy Foods

Carbohydrates provide us with calories for energy. Carbohydrate foods are starches, sugars, fats and proteins. They give the body varying degrees of energy, some more than others. The carbohydrates of natural foods are accompanied by micronutrients necessary for helping them to be utilized by the body. They give health and high energy. By contrast, the carbohydrates in overcooked, chemically treated, artificially flavored and colored processed foods (junk foods) contain so few micronutrients they have to rob the body of vitamins, minerals and enzymes to be utilized. As a result the bodies of junk food eaters are deficient. These people's health is in jeopardy. Highs that follow drain away leaving them tired, irritable and possibly discouraged or depressed. Here are list of foods and what they do for us. To keep energy up, eat high energy foods.

High Energy Foods That Give Health (Good)

Raw Nuts and seeds

Fresh, raw vegetables

Fresh, raw fruit

Homemade salad dressings of lemon juice, oil and vinegar, pureed avocado and nut and seed creams

Whole grain breads without preservatives or homemade breads; whole grain quick breads with no sugar

Whole grain crackers such as WASA bread and Zweibach, all without cooking oil or fat

Raw vegetable sticks, cherry tomatoes, crackers made of sprouted, dehydrated grains

Fresh fruits, sun-dried fruits, dried fruit cookies, raw fruit cakes or fruit ice creams (See recipes in the *UNcook Book* and *Bandwagon to Health.*)

Medium/Low Energy Foods Offering Little to Health (Fair)

Dry roasted nuts and seeds

Slightly steamed fresh vegetables

Frozen or slightly cooked fruits

Homemade dressings of yogurt, spiced oil and vinegar, mayonnaise without artificial ingredients, dressings without preservatives

"Wheat" breads made with white flour and bran or some cracked wheat; honey bran muffins

Whole grain crackers with cooking fat

Popcorn, cocoa milk (honey-sweetened), honey oatmeal cookies, unsweetened dry cereal, whole grain crackers made with oil

Cooked fruits, custards, whole wheat cakes, pies, cookies sweetened with date sugar, condensed frozen apple juice or honey

Low or No Energy Foods That May Destroy Health (Bad)

Roasted, oiled, salted nuts and seeds

Overcooked canned vegetables and sauces, such as catsup, relishes

Fruits canned in heavy syrup, candied or preserved

Commercial dressings containing artificial color, flavor, preservatives and synthetic, nutritionless ingredients

White bread (fifteen percent of nutrition of whole wheat), white flour, sugar sweet muffins, white biscuits, and breakfast sweet rolls containing sugar and caffeine

White flour crackers, salted; artificially colored cheese crackers with cooking fat and preservatives

Candy bars, cookies (sugar-containing), "juice drinks" potato chips, pretzels, sugared cereals, bakery goods, snack packs of crackers, processed cheese, sulphured dried fruits

Conventional cakes, pies, ice creams, pastries, candies, confections, doughnuts

Supplements: To Take or Not To Take?

A polluted world, foods grown on worn out, mineral depleted soil and the use of additives in processing those foods has led to universal deficiencies in people. It is becoming increasingly difficult to get sufficient nourishment for optimal health in foods alone. Millions turn to supplements. Yet how adequate are these supplements?

Reams have been written to answer this question. We will not attempt to resolve the controversy they have created. We wish only to alert the reader to some facts that have arisen in recent research and in our own experience.

We have found the *all natural food supplements* to be superior to vitamin or mineral or other nutrient substances prepared in a formula and offered as pills or capsules. If any of those preparations has as little as five percent natural ingredients, they can be labeled "natural." The rest, as in the case of vitamins, is apt to be synthetic. And the majority of the hundreds of people we have tested kinesiologically test weak on synthetic vitamins. People are often more harmed than helped by them.

Inorganic minerals in supplement preparations are frequently inefficiently utilized by the body. Chelated minerals are better. In these minerals, the molecule is grabbed onto by some nutrient or nutrients from plant sources, which helps them to be utilized much more efficiently. Enzymes are usually from an animal source and are more readily utilized by the body. However, they have a preservative which some are allergic to.

Nutrition-loaded foods are infinitely more effective in righting the wrong suffered from deficiencies. Their nutrients are in balance. They "treat" the whole body by supplying all its needs. They have no harmful side effects if the person isn't allergic to them. They cost *much* less. And you may not have to pay high consultation fees to learn to "balance" the minerals, the vitamins, and the enzymes if you eat a wide variety of natural foods. Here are some recommended high-nutrient foods:

Primary food yeast (cultured on molasses)
Torula yeast (cultured on wood pulp; has no selenium)
Brewers yeast
Spirulina plankton
Blue-green Algae
Wheat grass juice and (of late) powder
Barley grass juice and powder
Oat bran
Rice bran
Wheat germ (no more than a week old)
Bee pollen
Bee propolis
Royal jelly (contains natural preservatives to which some are allergic)
Sprouts of seeds, legumes, cereal grains, nuts
Kelp and other edible sea plants

The Beauties of Wheat Grass

The so-called fad for eating wheat grass is actually a custom that has been around for nearly 5,000 years. The ancient Greeks, Romans and Chinese all used it and paid great tribute to its curative powers. And for good reason.

From the soil wheat takes most of the 102 known minerals. (Its roots may go down nearly 100 feet.) This makes it one of the best of foods for day-to-day eating. It is also excellent for storage for survival. Seven-day-old wheat grass is full of minerals, enzymes and vitamins, especially vitamins C and A, B12, D, E, K, and U, and of course all the other known B vitamins. It is a complete food—proteins, carbohydrates, fats—with enzymes and chlorophyll in such abundance that, as far as is known, it is second only to corn which holds the record to date for "liquid sunshine," as many call it.

The ancients knew the efficacy of wheat grass for the maintenance of health and curing of diseases. The modern scientists have researched it in laboratories to find the reasons for that effectiveness—especially since Dr. Melvin Calvin's extensive and inspired research on the chemical reactions that would be produced by the plant in the presence of light energy, such as sunlight, electric light, or any light energy. His research and findings resulted in his receiving the Nobel Prize in 1962.

Interestingly, scientists have found that the chlorophyll molecule has the same structure as the hemoglobin (red blood cell) molecule. The difference between the two molecules is this: the center of the chlorophyll molecule is magnesium and the center of the hemoglobin molecule is iron.

The uses of wheat grass juice for nutrition and therapy are many. We list some of them here.

1. Wheat grass taken internally (an ounce or two one to three times a day, thirty minutes to an hour before meals) purifies the blood; detoxifies the body; helps to eliminate mucous in the intestines; helps chelate (take out) poisonous minerals such as lead, mercury and cadmium; improves energy, endurance, and general health; especially helps anemia; restores gray hair to original color; is effective against eczema and psoriasis, and helps reduce blood pressure. It also helps dissolve scar tissue, both externally (rubbed on) and internally; increases

hormonal activity; helps heal burns; aids in elevating constipation; nourishes the brain and nervous system; inhibits growth of cancer cells; prevents degenerative disease; improves the quality of cells; and acts as a restorer of body and mind.

2. Wheat grass juice used in the various orifices of the body is highly beneficial. It is so healing it can be used as a mouthwash, throat gargle, sinus irrigator or an eye or ear wash. Wheat grass juice can be used as a vaginal douche or as an implant after a high, water enema. Wait at least twenty minutes then put four to six ounces of freshly extracted wheat grass juice in the enema bag and proceed to place it in the rectum as you would an enema. Be sure you are lying down. Hold the wheat grass juice for twenty or thirty minutes, then expel. For complete directions, read *Be Your Own Doctor* by Dr. Ann Wigmore. (See Bibliography)

3. Wheat grass topical uses are many. Since the skin readily absorbs what is put on it, wheat grass is very effective rubbed in as a scalp tonic before a shampoo; as a sterilizer/healer on a sore or wound; as a skin cleanser; as a facial; and as nutrition when rubbed twenty times on the skin. Very ill persons can be nourished (fed) through the skin. Wheat grass also relieves an aching tooth and canker sores (hold pulp on affected part).

4. Wheat grass juice is invaluable in surviving radiation exposure; it increases resistance to X-rays; it helps protect one against the cell destruction of X-rays when used before they are taken; it slows down the harmful effects of air pollution and poisonous gasses such as carbon monoxide.

5. Other uses of wheat grass: When traveling, take along a cellophane bag of wheat grass and chew a handful now and then, spitting out the pulp. To help protect viewers from the radiation given off by color television, place a cafeteria tray or pan of growing wheat grass in front of set. Wheat grass growing in the house cleanses and deodorizes the air. A few blades of wheat grass defluorinates water, according to tests made by the New York City Water Department. Children grow and develop better and older people's cells are rejuvenated when taking wheat grass juice.

6. A word of warning on the use of wheat grass juice. While it has been repeatedly established that there is nothing toxic in wheat grass, the juice can cause nausea or a stomach ache when taken at first. One should start with only a teaspoonful and increase up to two ounces three times a day. You may want to dilute with equal amounts of fermec or water at first, and sip slowly, mixing well with the saliva. The philosophy, "If a little is good, more is better," does not apply to wheat grass juice. It is a powerful food and must be taken in respectful moderation.

7. Chlorophyll Green Drinks can be delicious. They give a lovely "high" without any depressing "lows." Here are a few recipes to inspire your own creativity:

Celery-Wheat Grass
 5 oz celery juice
 1 oz wheat grass juice
 1 oz distilled water

*Wheat Grass Pineappleade**
 4 oz pineapple juice
 2 oz wheat grass juice
 1 to 2 oz distilled water

Dr. Baker's Green Green Drink
 2 oz comfrey juice
 2 oz celery juice
 1 to 2 oz wheat grass juice

Vegetable Juice Cocktail
 3 oz carrot
 2 oz celery
 1 oz fermec
 1 or 2 oz wheat grass juice

Favorite Green Drink
 2 1/2 oz wheat grass juice
 2 or 3 oz fermec

*Lemon Green**
   2 oz wheat grass juice
   1 oz lemon juice
   1 or 2 teaspoons honey
   4 oz distilled water

*Recommended only occasionally. Wheat grass is a vegetable and doesn't mix well with fruits.

Deadly Don'ts

Foods that have been changed from their original state fresh out of the field, garden or orchard can be harmful because the body not only can't utilize them, it can't eliminate them the way it does waste from natural foods. These altered substances are foreign and act as toxins, poisoning the bloodstream and system. This contributes to degenerative disease and premature aging.

Following is a list of "do not eats" with a word about why.

Refined Sugar—Beyond giving the eater a spurt of energy, it only does harm. It is a carbohydrate without nutrition. Sugar is as addictive as drugs. It robs the body of vitamins and minerals, upsets the metabolism, causes wide mood and energy swings, plus irritability and poor memory.

Fats, Margarine (processed vegetable oils, beef and pork)—In the hydrogenation process, the polyunsaturated oils (linoleic acid and linolenic acid) are chemically altered and cannot be utilized as food by the body. They end up as sticky plaque on the walls of the arteries; cholesterol sticks to that plaque. Margarines not only are hydrogenated, they have artificial flavor and artificial color, both toxins.

When fats are heated to frying and broiling temperatures, they are indigestible. Especially undesirable are fats used to deep fry over and over in restaurants and fast food outlets. They are one of the greatest contributors to heart disease, constipation, varicose veins and obesity.

White Flour—Eighty-five percent of the nutrition is removed with the germ and hull of the wheat grain! That means most of the minerals, B vitamins and vitamin E are also removed. The nearly worthless white flour is then "enriched" with inorganic iron that the body does not utilize and some synthetic B vitamin to which most people are allergic. There aren't enough trace nutrients left for it to be utilized by the body.

Coffee, Tea, Cola Drinks—Caffeine is a stimulant. It is addictive. It destroys vitamin C and other vitamins in the body. Taken as hot coffee or tea, it inhibits digestion in the stomach and can cause the beginning of ulcers. Colas not only contain sugar or artificial sweeteners, they have artificial color, are ice cold (thus unnatural) for the stomach, contain carbonization causing an "explosion" in the stomach, and take the place of nutritious foods in satisfying the appetite and the need for water to quench thirst. Colas are all bad.

Alcohol—Alcohol is a vitamin robber; it is addictive. It causes severe vitamin deficiencies and cravings for more alcohol and sugar.

Chemically Loaded Foods—Artificial flavors, artificial colors, preservatives, some emulsifiers and extenders, bleaches, and synthetic (artificial) foods rob us of health. They are toxic and toxins torture the body, the nervous system and the brain.

Salt—Salt is necessary to the body, not to the appetite. Our appetite for excessive salt is cultivated by eating processed foods. Natural foods contain natural salt in sufficient quantity unless the soil they were grown in was salt deficient, as in the Pacific Northwest. Too much salt is truly deadly. Yet too little salt puts potassium out of balance, causes fatigue and contributes to low blood pressure. The little bit of salt that may be needed should be unprocessed sea salt.

Body pH Chart

```
                                                    8.0
                                              7.5
                                        7.0
                                  6.5
                            6.0
                      5.5
                5.0
          4.5

     Acid       Normal Range      Neutral       Alkaline
```

pH is the letter symbol for the acid-alkaline balance of the body. The range is indicated by numbers from 4.5 to 8.0.

You can test for body pH by running a little urine of the first morning voiding over a piece of nitrozene paper bought at any drugstore. The determination is made by matching the color with the small chart on the package. 4.5 is canary yellow. 6.0 is green. 7.0 or 7.5 is deep purple. 8.0 is purplish black.

In the 1960's, doctors observed that "normal" pH for the body was not 7.0 or neutral, but somewhere near 6.0. With further clinical observation they began to realize optionally healthy persons often had a pH of 5.0 or 5.5 and anything more alkaline indicated a less vigorous state of health.

In observing our health, we notice when we bounce out of bed in the morning feeling joyous, close to the Lord and ready for any challenge, our first voiding pH is 5.0 or 5.5, without exception. When we get up feeling dragged out and a bit reluctant to face the day, our pH is 6.5 or 7.0.

The reason? When the body is functioning optimally, the immune system is doing its work and the body is protected from illness by one of its greatest defenses, a slightly acid condition.

What's so great about being slightly acid? Bacteria and virus cannot proliferate in an acid environment. A slightly acid mantle of the skin, our largest organ, protects us from unimaginable hosts of microbes in the environment. We do not live in a sterilized world. The strong hydrochloric acid of the stomach protects us from all sorts of microbes, amoeba and parasites.

How do we get our pH from alkaline to slightly acid? Prunes,

apple cider vinegar, cranberry juice, blueberries and hydrochloric acid (betaine hydrochloride or glutamic acid hydrochloride) will quickly help. The body pH will slowly right itself
on an all-natural, mainly raw eating regime without the extra
acid in the above. Animal flesh and eggs help the nonvegetarian
to an acid pH. Many heavy meat eaters have too low a pH—4.0
to 4.5. They're not susceptible to colds and flu but they may have
more serious long range diseases.

Dr. William A. Ellis, a physician friend who practiced
nutritional medicine for nearly forty years, says that all people
with infections, cancer and general ill health have a high pH.
Our experience confirms this.

Kinesiology Testing for Adults:

The Kinesiology Test for allergies, or muscle strength test,
has come of age. It is quick. It costs nothing. And, as several
physicians have remarked, it is amazingly unerring! Discovered
and developed by Dr. George Goodheart and further researched
by such scientists as John Diamond, M.D., it is being used by
physicians, dentists, osteopaths, chiropractors, naturopaths and
other therapists. If carefully done, closely following instructions, responsible adults can test each other for food and
materials allergies.

To do the testing, follow these instructions: The subject to be
tested stands and extends his or her arm and hand straight out
from and level with the shoulder. The person who does the
testing (the tester), with one hand on the subject's wrist, pulls
down on the extended arm, while the subject resists as much as
possible.

Keeping in mind the strength felt in the extended arm, the
tester then puts some object like a banana in the subject's left
hand. Again the subject extends the right arm and makes it
rigid. Again the tester pulls down on the arm. If it is more easily
pulled down than in the trial test of strength, the subject is
allergic to bananas. His body is weakened by contact with the
banana that is known to be toxic. For maximum strength and
freedom from the fatigue factor, he should avoid bananas.

A double check can be made on the banana. The subject
presses the end of the little finger to the end of the thumb of the
left hand with all the strength that can be applied. The tester
tries to pull the finger and thumb apart, grasping each at the last

joint, thus testing the strength of the subject's hand. Now the tester places the banana in the right hand while the subject presses together the thumb and little finger of the left. The tester tries to pull the thumb and finger apart. If done so fairly easily (as against pulling them apart with great difficulty before), the subject's body is allergic to bananas.

The test was conducted on one patient by another patient in the presence of the doctor who taught us how to do the testing. Here's what the doctor had patients John and Mike do. John was the tester, Mike the subject.

1. Mike extended his right arm straight out from his shoulder, his fist clenched, his arm rigid.
2. John tested the strength of Mike's arm by pulling down on it at the wrist after he said, "Resist me." This showed John how much strength was in Mike's arm. He had to exert considerable effort to pull Mike's arm down.
3. Into Mike's left hand, relaxed at his side, was placed a polyester sock.
4. Mike again made his extended right arm rigid and clenched his fist to resist Johns trying to pull it down.
5. John had little trouble pulling Mike's arm down this time. Mike's body was weakened by contact with the polyester, a toxic material. In the present day parlance, Mike was "allergic" to polyester.

To double-check the result of the test, the doctor taught John and Mike the other way to do the same test.

1. Mike pressed the tip of his little finger to the tip of his thumb of his right hand as hard as he could. His empty left hand was relaxed at his side.
2. With difficulty, John pulled the thumb and finger apart. Mike had formidable strength in his fingers.
3. Mike again received the polyester sock in his left hand while he pressed his right finger and thumb together.
4. John pulled Mike's little finger and thumb apart with minimum effort.
5. Again Mike's strength was weakened by contact with polyester.

The doctor gave two small objects to John to do another test on Mike, this time a blind test.

1. Mike extended his arm.
2. John tested the strength in Mike's arm by grasping the wrist and pulling down on it. There was formidable strength in the arm.
3. Into Mike's left hand, held palm up, slightly back of him and out of his sight, John laid the two small objects.
4. Mike again made his arm rigid and clenched his fist to resist John's testing of his strength.
5. John had little trouble pulling Mike's arm down.

The doctor then showed Mike the two vitamin tablets John had laid in Mike's hand, vitamins the doctor thought of prescribing. But with Mike's body showing an allergic response, the doctor, of course, did not prescribe them.

The doctor had John test Mike on kelp tablets, this time using the finger-thumb method. Mike was deficient in several minerals and the doctor wanted not only to know if Mike was allergic to kelp, but how many tablets he should take. He cautioned John to be very careful in assessing Mike's strength before testing the kelp. This test could have been done blind but the doctor chose to have it done open, using the little finger-to-thumb method.

1. Mike pressed his little finger to his thumb (right hand).
2. John had difficulty pulling them apart.
3. John put one kelp tablet in Mike's left hand.
4. Mike again pressed his finger against his thumb.
5. John found the strength in Mike's hand unchanged.
6. John put another kelp tablet in Mike's hand and found the strength in Mike's thumb and finger greater.
7. John put the third tablet in Mike's left hand and found even greater strength in the thumb-pressed-against-finger on the right hand.
8. John put the fourth kelp tablet in Mike's left hand and could hardly pull the thumb and finger of the right hand apart, so great was the strength.
9. John placed the fifth kelp tablet in Mike's left hand and found that the finger-thumb pressure of the right hand was weak.

Thus according to his "body language message," the proper dosage of kelp for Mike was four tablets (taken with meals).

John did a few more tests on Mike, part of the time using Mike's left arm or hand for the strength testing. (In testing several things at one session, alternate the hand and arm used for strength-testing to avoid undue tiring.)

Later at home, the two young men continued the testing at intervals. Mike's favorite vegetables were corn and peas, but he had noticed that he felt sluggish after eating peas. When John did a blind test of the two vegetables by laying a few of first one then the other in Mike's palm, he found that the strength in Mike's hand and arm was greatly diminished when holding the peas.

Mike learned through Kinesiology Testing that he was allergic to peas, peanuts, cooked starches (cereal, grains, potatoes, rice, mango, lamb, beef, pork, chicken and turkey, plus such over-the-counter drugs as aspirin and antacid, and his favorite brand of toothpaste. He was allergic to scented soap and household cleansers, polyethylene (car upholstery) and synthetic rubber, besides the polyester and soft plastics. By eliminating all those things in his home, he feels great and is over the illnesses he suffered as the result of his many allergies and sensitivities. With his much improved health and diet, he is able to tolerate the everyday toxins he encounters away from home if not exposed to them for too long a time.

Anyone can learn to conduct these tests, provided common sense and a few guidelines are observed. The Kinesiology Test for allergies is not a parlor game. It is a serious, highly useful test for indicating why the body may be suffering from weakness, dysfunction, fatigue or illness. Here are a few things to keep in mind while testing:

* Do the testing in private, free from distraction.
* Plan to test only a few things at a session.
* Do not continue testing after the subject is found to be allergic to something. The fatigue of the arm or finger-thumb sometimes carries over to another test and affects the results.
* Even though the subject does not test allergic, he or she should not be tested on more than three things in a row because the fatigue in the arm and/or hand may alter the test results.

* Testing is best done by adult members of the family or close friends.
* In the case of an ill person, test only one thing at a session. The thumb-finger test is advisable.
* If the subject tires, he or she should lightly tap three or four times over the thymus gland, about three inches below the center dip in the collar bone, to restore strength.
* If the food or object to be tested cannot be held by the hand of the subject, the hand can be placed against or on top of it.
* Gases can be tested by having the subject breathe fresh air during the preliminary appraisal of the strength of arm and fingers. Afterward, he breathes the gas as the strength of his fingers or arm is tested.

Note: *Both the tester and the subject must remain serious during the testing. Smiling alters results.*

Before anyone can prescribe a proper diet, he or she needs to know what foods may cause a problem. If a food causes a sensitivity (allergy), that food becomes a poison that the system has to cope with. If the liver is healthy and can detoxify the unusable food, no particular problem is noted. But if the liver cannot detoxify the offending food, the body has a problem which may show up as indigestion, grogginess, headache, constipation, skin condition, arthritis and so on.

Use the Kinesiology Test carefully to reveal offending foods. The body does not lie. Avoid eating food that cuts the body's energy as indicated by the test. After a few weeks, try eating the food all alone if you do not have full confidence in the test and see if you feel good after eating it. If not, you know to leave it alone.

About every six months, we retest a food that we were sensitive to. Once in awhile, we find one that no longer gives a problem. In such a case, we eat it only periodically.

In theory, the body should not be sensitive to any foods if it is receiving optimal nutrition. However, in our present society there are many extenuating circumstances that alter our food requirements. There are pollutants that may cause us to need more vitamins. Also, each person may need different amounts of certain nutrients in different combinations. No two of us are alike. The human body is a marvelous, extremely complicated mechanism. Science does not yet know why some can eat a perfectly good, highly nutritious, pure, natural food and some can't. But the body will tell us if we consult it. Remember that it tells the truth. Follow the rules and use the Kinesiology Test to know that truth.

Children's Kinesiology Testing

A child anywhere from infancy to twelve years old can be accurately tested for food allergies by using an adult surrogate, such as the mother. The father or another responsible adult acts as the tester. So there are three people: the child to be tested, the surrogate and the tester. (In the case of a baby, a fourth person is needed to hold the infant's hand containing the food or substance being tested.)

Have the child stand up. Lay the infant on it's back on a table. The surrogate stands next to the child or infant with her left hand on the back of the subject's neck. The tester tests the right arm of the surrogate for its strength. Then the surrogate gently taps his/her thymus area (two and one half to three inches below the little dip in the collar bone) a time or two. The tester tests the strength of the surrogate's arm again, making a mental note of its maximum strength.

A piece of wheat bread is placed in the child's hand with the surrogate's left hand on the subject's neck. Again the tester tests the strength of the surrogate's arm. It may be the same, stronger or weaker. If the arm is weaker, that food (bread) does not give the child energy. It takes away from his energy. Eating that food weakens the child's defenses and helps to make him more vulnerable to disease. It should be totally eliminated.

In this way a child can be tested for every kind of food, for all drinks (a teaspoon of liquid held in the palm of the hand), for synthetic fabrics, for household cleaning products, for medications, for everything. Not until all allergen containing foods, water, liquids and substances are removed and a nourishing diet of all natural, mostly raw foods provided, can the child hope to have vigorous optimal health.

Hypoglycemia Symptoms

Hypoglycemia, commonly called low blood sugar, plagues the western world. Estimates of the percentage of people in the United States with low blood sugar run from forty to seventy percent of the population. It is found in all ages, small children included. Our nutrition robbed diet of processed foods and drinks is largely to blame.

We list below symptoms of hypoglycemia that some alternate therapy doctors have recorded. We experienced many of them before we discovered our allergies and "cleaned up" our diet. You can check which ones apply to you. If you are one of the thousands who are ill and for whom no other cause has been diagnosed, you will know to suspect hypoglycemia.

Headache
Tiredness without cause
Fast heart palpitations
Constant hunger
Sweating without cause
Allergy prone
Nervousness
Limited sex drive (impotence, frigidity)
Stomach gas
Confusion
Depression
Lack of coordination
Indigestion
Sudden weight loss or gain
Drowsiness
Poor concentration
Unconsciousness
Motion sickness
Constipation
Asthma
Ulcers
Cold feet and hands
Arthritic pains
Speech difficulties
Obesity
Insomnia
Poor memory

Angina
Hyperactivity
Mental deficiency
Lack of appetite
Restlessness
Convulsions
Alcoholism
Vision problems (double vision, blurred or dimness of vision)
Craving for (addiction) sugar, cigarettes, soft drinks, caffeine, drugs
Nightmares
Sleepiness
Muscle pain
Fainting
Suicidal tendencies
Heartburn
Antisocial behavior
Irritability
Disturbed and intermittent sleep
Stumbling or loss of muscle control
High blood pressure
Low blood pressure
Narcolepsy
Frequent tonsillitis especially in children
Schizophrenia and personality changes
Paranoia
Food addiction (allergies)
Phobias, fears
Slow learning
Epilepsy
Mood swings
Dizziness
Crying spells
Neurosis, psychosis
Tremors, inside flutters
Cold, clammy skin
Numbness, tingling in hands, feet
Gasping for breath
Anxiety
Juvenile delinquency
Weakness
Heavy sighing

Needless worry
Restless legs

Exercises of the Astronauts

These exercises are effective for tension in the neck and base of the head, for helping to relax the whole body, for clearer thinking and greater mental efficiency. They can be done by almost everyone including ill people, shut-ins and the aged. Additionally, they can be reduced or increased to fit the need and done almost anywhere at any time. The single, most effective set of exercises we do, they help to keep us feeling good and thinking well.

Neck and base of head exercises can be done either sitting erect in a straight chair or standing barefoot or in flat heeled shoes. Arms should be limp and relaxed at the sides of the body, shoulders straight, head up.

1. Let the head fall forward as though the neck were cooked spaghetti. Roll the head to one shoulder, on around to the back, then the other shoulder, then back to the beginning position. Repeat this head roll or circle exercise a total of three times returning to the head-erect position.

2. With the head still erect, back straight, lift shoulders high (arms hanging limp), then push them back as far as possible, then let them drop. Repeat at total of three times. Enjoy the relaxed feeling for a few moments.

3. With mouth closed slowly tilt head back and hold to a moderately slow count of ten (ten seconds). Then slowly tilt the head forward, all the way, until the chin is resting on the chest. Hold to a count of ten. Repeat two more times.

4. Hunch shoulders high, lean the head back against them, pressing hard, and turn from left to right in a relaxing self massage. Do this about ten times.

5. Push the crown of the head up as high as possible, holding to a count of ten. Relax.

6. Imagine a string attached to your right ear and pulling it up high. Hold in this position for ten counts. Repeat with the left ear, then relax.

7. Push your head up and out (it's called turtle-necking)
    while opening your mouth wide and sticking you tongue
    out as far as possible. Hold to a count of ten. Relax with
    the mouth closed.

Measurement/Equivalent Tables

1,000,000	micrograms	(mcg.)	= 1 milligram
1,000	milligrams	(mg.)	= 1 gram
1,000	grams	(gr.)	= 1 kilogram
1	kilogram	(kilo)	= 2 pounds, 2 ounces
1/4	teaspoon		= approximately 1 gram (as in vitamin C powder
3	teaspoons		= 1 tablespoon
4	tablespoons		= 1/4 cup = 2 ounces
8	tablespoons		= 1/2 cup = 4 ounces
2	cups		= 1 pint
2	pints		= 1 quart
4	quarts		= 1 gallon

Part VI

Directory of Products, Sources and Services

Listed below are organic food growers, manufacturers, associations and businesses offering useful services and products. They are here for the sole purpose of helping our readers. We receive no financial compensation, nor have we any connection with them. Please write to them directly for further information.

American College of Advancement in Medicine (ACAM). 6151 W. Century Blvd., Suite 1114, Los Angeles, CA 90045 (One of their goals is to insure public awareness of alternative holistic methods of prevention and treatment. Physician membership directory is $3.50.)

Bronson Pharmaceuticals. 4526 Rinetti Lane, La Canada, CA 91011–0628 (Powdered vitamin C as ascorbic acid, calcium ascorbate; other vitamin products; minerals.)

Cancer Control Society. 2043 N. Berendo St., Los Angeles, CA 90026.

Deva Natural Clothes, Box S86, Burkittsville, MD 21718

Diamond K Enterprises, R.R. 1, Box 30, St. Charles, MN 55972 (Organic food products.)

Ecology Sound Farms, Norman Freestone, 42126 Road 168, Orosi, CA 93647 (Organic foods.)

Feingold Association of the United States, Drawer AG, Holts-ville, NY 11742 (Information on hyperactivity.)

Good Food Company, 319 Riverside Ct., Kent, OH 44240 (Natural, whole foods.)

Great Date in the Morning, P.O. Box 31, Coachella, CA 92236 (Organic foods, especially dried fruits.)

Healthier Children/Happier Futures. % Susan Barnett, Forest Hill Road, Dunstable, MA 01827.

Juice Suite, P.O. Box 701, Bloomfield, CT 06002 (Grass juicers, blenders and vegetable juicers; discount on many of the appliances. Send fifty cents for information and price list.)

Lee Anderson's Covalda Date Co., P.O. Box 908, Coachella, CA 92236

Living Farms, Box 50, Tracy, MN 56175 (Organic farm products.)

Moullinex (Spice and coffee grinder which is made in France, typically available in health food stores.)

National Health Federation. P.O. Box 688, Monrovia, CA 91016 (The largest organization fighting for health freedoms.)

Natural Development Co., Bainbridge, PA 17502 (Cress seeds, sunflower seeds, buckwheat, lentils, corn, wheat, alfalfa. Free postage east of the Mississippi River. Free catalog.)

Oak Manner Milling, Rural Route 1, Tavistock, Ontario, Canada, N0B 2R0 (Whole grains and flour.)

Organic Farm & Garden Center, Box 2806, San Rafael, CA 94901

Plastaket Manufacturing, 6226 Highway 12, Lodi, CA 95240 (Champion food processor.)

Shiloh Farms, Rt. 59, Sulphur Springs, AR 72768 (Ask for price list of seeds and foods.)

Sundance Industries, 28 Vermont Ave., White Plains, NY 10606 (Their Wheatena model "S" is an ideal juicer for wheat grass and a grinder for sprouted grains.)

Timber Crest Farms, 4791 Dry Creek Road, Healdsburg, CA 95448 (Organic foods, grains, seeds and other products.)

Vita Mix, 8615 Usher Rd., Cleveland, OH 44138 (Model 3600 is excellent as a blender and grain or seed grinder.)

Walnut Acres, Pennscreek, PA 17862. (Grains, seeds, granolas. Lots of natural foods, kitchen appliances and equipment. Catalog available.)

Glossary

ACTH (adrenocorticotropia hormone): a polypeptide hormone produced by the anterior lobe of the pituitary gland which stimulates the cortical substance of human adrenal glands; Pharmaceutical: This substance is extracted from the pituitary glands of hogs and other species, in the form of its white water-soluble powder, and used in the treatment of rheumatic fever, rheumatoid arthritis and various allergic disorders.

Acupuncture: a traditional practice in Chinese folk medicine of striving to cure illness by puncturing specified areas of the skin with needles.

Acidophilus: a fermented milk produced by growing the bacterium Lactobacillus acidophilus in milk, used in medicine to alter the microbial flora of the intestinal tract under certain conditions; often referred to as the "good" flora.

Addison's Disease: a disease characterized by asthenia, low blood pressure, and a brownish skin coloration, due to disturbance of the suprarenal glands; atrophy of the adrenal glands.

Agoraphobia: an abnormal fear of being in an open space.

Aldosterone: a hormone produced by the cortex of the adrenal gland, instrumental in the regulation of sodium and potassium reabsorption by the cells of the tubular portion of the kidney. This hormone helps to hold necessary salt in the tissues.

Amino acids: any of a class of organic compounds that contains at least one carboxyl group and one amino group.

Antihistamines: any of certain compounds or medicines that neutralize or inhibit the effect of histamine in the body. Used chiefly in the treatment of allergic disorders and colds.

Antioxidants: any substance inhibiting oxidation; the destruction of oxygen.

Antiviral: the opposite of viral. In medicine, something that works against, inhibits, kills, or destroys ultramicroscopic, infectious agents called virus.

Arginase: enzyme the body produces to metabolize the amino acid arginine.

Arginine: one of the essential amino acids that make up plant and animal proteins.

Arteriosclerosis: an arterial disease occurring especially in the elderly. Characterized by inelasticity and thickening of the vessel walls, with lessened blood flow.

Atherosclerosis: a form of arteriosclerosis in which fatty substances deposit in and beneath the intima, which is the lining of the arteries.

Autolysis: the destruction of cells of the body by its own serum; also called *autocytolysis*. Postmortem autolysis: enzymatic self-destruction of cells or tissues after death.

Betaine hydrochloride: a form of hydrochloric acid (stomach acid) used medicinally for deficiency of stomach acid, necessary to digest proteins.

Binders: substances used to hold together the ingredients of a pill or tablet.

Bioflavonoid complex: the vitamin C complex.

Caffeine: a white, crystalline, bitter alkaloid usually derived from coffee or tea; used in medicine as a stimulant or diuretic. Also used in bakery goods to enhance the flavor.

Carcinogenic: a substance that tends to produce cancer.

Cholecystectomy: surgical procedure used to remove the gall bladder.

Colitis: inflammation of the colon.

Corticosteroids: any of a class of steroids, as aldosterone, hydrocortisone, or cortisone, occurring in nature as a product of the adrenal cortex, or synthesized.

Deleterious: injurious to health.

Dementia: severe impairment or loss of intellectual capacity and personality integration.

Detrusor muscle: a muscle that has an outward or downward thrust or force.

Diuretics: drugs, or natural foods such as watermelon, that help the body rid itself of water retention.

EDTA: (edetate) ethylenediaminotetraaceetate. Any salt of edetic acid; a metal chelating agent used in the diagnosis, treatment and removal of lead and other heavy metal poisoning; and because of its affinity for calcium in the treatment of hypercalcemia.

Emphysema: abnormal distension of an organ or a part of the body, especially the lungs, with air or other gas.

Entero-vioform: a powerful drug used some years ago especially for such infestations, as amoeba and other parasites. Side reactions from taking the drug were found to be so deleterious it is now rarely used.

Enzymes: complex organic substances within the body and in plants, as pepsin, originating from living cells and capable of producing chemical changes in organic substances—as in digestion. Examples are the enzyme plytin, produced in the mouth from chewing food, necessary to stimulate the production of hydrochloric acid in the stomach and pancreatic enzymes to aid in further digestion of foods in the small intestine.

Esophagitis: inflammation of the esophagus.

Flaxseed: the seed of flax, historically called the seeds of the linen plant.

Fungal Dermatitis: a moldlike skin fungus.

Gastroenteritis: inflammation of the stomach and intestines.

Gastrointestinal tract: the entire digestive system from the throat to the anus—esophagus, stomach, duodenum, small intestine and large intestine (colon).

Glutamic acid: an amino acid used chiefly in the form of sodium salt as a seasoning.

Glycogen: body starch synthesized by the liver.

Gram: a metric unit. One thousandth of a kilogram. Approximately one fourth teaspoon.

Hard soaps: soaplike deposits in the intestines formed from undigested fats and highly alkaline food substances.

Hesperidin: a bioflavonoid glycoside occurring in most citrus fruits, especially in the spongy envelope of oranges and lemons.

Histidine: a basic amino acid converted by putrefactive organisms into histamine.

Histamine: an amine compound released in allergic reactions. It dilates blood vessels, stimulates gastric secretions, and causes contraction of the uterus.

Horsetail: (also called shave grass) a medicinal herb very high in digestible silicon. Found to be effective in recovery from osteoporosis.

Hydrogen peroxide: a solution used as an antiseptic and a bleaching agent. Sometimes prescribed by physicians in a diluted solution for getting more oxygen into the cells for better health and resistance to disease.

Hyperactive: unusually or excessively active.

Hypertension: excessive or extreme tension.

Hypochlorhydria: deficiency of stomach acid (hydrochloric acid).

Hypoglycemia: an abnormally low level of glucose in the blood.

Hypothyroidism: deficient activity of the thyroid gland.

Iatrogenic: caused by the diagnosis, manner, or treatment, especially drugs, of a physician or surgeon.

Inflammation: redness, swelling, pain, tenderness, heat, and disturbed function of an area of the body, especially as a reaction of tissues to injurious agents.

Interferon: a protein substance produced by virus-invaded cells that prevents reproduction of the virus.

Inositol: an essential growth factor for animal life. Widely distributed in plants and seeds and present in animal tissues, urine, and the vitamin B complex.

Intravenous: within a vein or veins. Pertaining to, employed in, or administered by an injection into the vein.

Irradiation: exposure, or the process of exposure to, X-rays or other radiation.

Kaposi's Sarcoma: a tumor made up of a substance like embryonic tissue; tissue composed of closely packed cells often highly malignant.

Kefir: a kind of milk culture similar to yogurt.

Legumes: any of a large family of herbs, shrubs, and trees, including the peas, beans, vetches, clovers, alfalfa, etc.

Lesion: an injury, hurt, or wound.

Lactobacillus acidophilus: (see acidophilus)

Lysine: a basic amino acid essential in the nutrition of humankind and animals.

Masticate: to chew well.

Megadose: very large doses.

Metabolism: the sum of the physical and chemical processes in an organism by which protoplasm is produced, maintained and destroyed, and by which energy is made available for its functioning.

Methionine: an amino acid found in casein, wool and other proteins or prepared synthetically. Used as a supplement to a high protein diet in the prevention and treatment of certain diseases and infections.

Microgram: a unit of weight equal to one millionth of a gram.

Milligram: a unit of weight equal to one thousandth of a gram.

Meniere's Disease: a disease of the inner ear which affects a person's balance.

Mitotic: referring to mitosis, the method or process of normal cell division.

Modality: a treatment. The application of a therapeutic agent, usually a physical therapeutic agent.

Motility: the capability of moving spontaneously.

Mucous: (also mucus) slimy, thick liquid or discharge.

Narcolepsy: an unnatural condition characterized by frequent and uncontrollable need for short periods of deep sleep.

Naturopathy: method of treating disease using food, herbs, exercise, heat, etc., to assist the natural healing processes.

Nucleic acid: any of a group of complex acids occurring in all living cells, especially as a component of cell-nucleus proteins, and composed of a phosphoric acid group, a carbohydrate, two purines, and two pyrimidines.

Nutritional: of or pertaining to nutrition, nourishment; the sustaining with food.

Nystatin: brand name for a type of antibiotic effective in the treatment and elimination of a yeast overgrowth in the body called Candida albicans.

Oleic acid: a water-insoluble liquid unsaturated acid used chiefly in the manufacture of soap and cosmetics.

Oncologist: a specialist in the detection and treatment of tumors.

Opnea: cessation of breathing; asphyxia.

Ophthalmologist: a physician specializing in treating problems and diseases of the eye; an eye specialist qualified to perform eye surgery.

Ornithine: an amino acid obtained by the hydrolysis of arginine.

Oropharynx: the part of the pharynx between the soft palate and the upper edge of the epiglottis.

Orthomolecular: referring to correct or healthy cells.

PABA (Para-aminobenzoic acid): a compound occurring in, and sometimes classified with, the B vitamins. Used chiefly in the manufacture of dyes and pharmaceuticals.

Pangamic Acid: vitamin B15.

Pantothenic acid: an oily, hydroxy acid found in plant and animal tissues, rice, bran, etc., and essential for cell growth. Classified as a B vitamin.

Petrochemicals: chemicals derived from petroleum.

Phagocytic: of or pertaining to phagocyte. A white blood cell. A blood cell that ingests and destroys foreign particles, bacteria and other cells.

Phospholipid: any of a group of fatty compounds as lecithin, composed of phosphoric esters, and occurring in cellular organisms.

Phytate: (phytic acid) a white to pale yellow, water-soluble liquid found in cereal grains. Used commercially as a water softener. Too much phytate in the diet can block the body's utilization of zinc, an essential trace mineral.

Plaque: a rubbery, tough, sticky substance that forms on the arterial walls from hydrogenated fats (oils and margarines). Also a gelatinous accumulation of bacteria and mucin that forms on teeth.

Polyps: a projecting growth from a mucous surface, as of the nose, being either a tumor or a hypertrophy of the mucous membrane.

Poi: a pastelike Hawaiian food made of the root of the taro plant which is baked, pounded, moistened, and fermented.

Process-depleted: terminology applied to foods so overprocessed they have few nutrients left in the finished product.

Psyllium husks: the hull or husk of psyllium, an edible seed valued for its cleansing (cathartic) effect in the bowels. Used as a food extender and thickener, and as extra bulk in the diet.

Purine: a compound from which is derived a group of substances including uric acid, xanthine, and caffeine.

Putrefaction: the process of rot or decay. The decomposition of organic matter by bacteria and fungi.

Pyrimidines: a heterocyclic ring compound that is an important constituent of several biochemical substances, as thiamine, which is vitamin B1.

Reflexology: a type of foot and hand massage, found by many to be effective in stimulating the organs of the body to action and to relieve pain and other symptoms.

Ribonucleic acid: RNA; one of the class of nucleic acids found chiefly in the cytoplasm of cells.

Ropy: stringy, mucilaginous, viscid.

Schizophrenia: psychosis marked by withdrawn, bizarre, sometimes disillusioned behavior and by intellectual and emotional deterioration.

Shave grass: see horsetail.

Sjogren's syndrome: a symptom complex of unknown etiology (knowledge regarding causes of disease) usually in middle-aged and older women in which inflammation of the cornea and conjunctiva are associated with dry mouth and throat, and enlargement of the parotid gland near the ear.

Silica: a mineral utilized by the body as calcium, or given for the prevention or correction of osteoporosis.

Spirulina plankton: fresh water edible algae, a complete food although vitamin C occurs in a small amount. A dark, bright green, it contains much of the healing factor chlorophyll. It also is the highest in B12, the antianemia factor, of any known food including liver, the second highest known food source.

Staphylococcus: any of several bacteria, certain species of which can be disease producing for humans.

Sticky plaque: see plaque.

Surrogate: one chosen to act for another.

Surrogate testing: Kinesiology Testing an adult who touches the subject (infant, child, athlete, or invalid) holding the food or substance being tested.

Synthesize: to combine (constituent elements) into a single or unified entity.

T4 cell count: one of several cell types produced by the thymus gland.

Tachycardia: excessively rapid heartbeat.

Taurine: a crystalline substance obtained from the bile of animals, used in biochemical research.

Tehini: a seed butter made of sesame seed meal and vegetable oil.

Therapist: a person trained in physical, psychological, or other therapy.

Topically: state or quality of being applied to a particular part of the body; locally.

Torula Yeast: an edible yeast, similar to brewers yeast but lacking in selenium. It is cultured on wood pulp.

Tryptophan: an essential amino acid occurring in the seeds of some leguminous plants. Released from proteins by tryptic digestion, and important in the nutrition of animals.

Urea: a compound occurring in urine and other body fluids as a product of protein metabolism.

Vagina: the passage leading from the uterus to the vulva in women.

Vaginitis: inflammation of the vagina.

Vermifuge: serving to expel worms or other animal parasites from the intestines, as a medicine.

Viral: of, pertaining to, or caused by virus.

Vitiligo: a skin disease characterized by smooth, white patches on various parts of the body, caused by the loss of the natural pigment.

Volatile: evaporating; passing off readily in the form of vapor.

Wheat grass juice implants: the juice of seven-day-old wheat grass placed in the rectum and colon by an enema syringe and bag, or special enema bucket, ten to twenty minutes after a water enema.

Bibliography

Airola, Paavo. *Health Secrets From Europe.* West Nyack, NY: Parker Publishing Company, Inc, 1970.

Airola, Paavo. *How To Get Well.* Phoenix, AZ: Health Plus Publishers, 1976.

Baker, Elizabeth and Baker, Dr. Elton. *The UNcook Book.* Portland, OR: Drelwood Publications, Distributed by Communication Creativity, 1980.

Baker, Elizabeth and Baker, Dr. Elton. *Bandwagon To Health.* Portland, OR: Drelwood Publications, Distributed by Communication Creativity, 1984.

Buckinger, Otto H.F. *About Fasting—A Royal Road To Healing.* Wellingborough, Northhamptonshire, England: Thorons Publishers Limited, 1976.

Carter, Albert E. *The Miracles of Rebound Exercise.* Snohomish, WA: Snohomish Publishing Co.,Inc., 1979.

Cott, Allen. *Fasting, The Ultimate Diet.* 1975.

Diamond, John, M.D. *Your Body Doesn't Lie.* New York, NY: Warner Books, Inc., 1979.

Dufty, William. *Sugar Blues.* New York, NY: Warner Books, Inc., 1975.

Feingold, Ben E. *Why Your Child Is Hyperactive.* Westminister, MD: Random House, 1985.

Fredericks, Carlton. *Psycho-Nutrition.* New York: Grosset & Dunlap, 1978.

Guthrie, Helen Andrews. *Introductory Nutrition*. Saint Louis, MO: The C.V. Mosby Company, 1975.

Gray, Robert. *The Colon Cleansing Handbook*. Oakland, CA: Rockbridge Publishing Co., 1982.

Illich, Ivan. *Medical Nemesis*. New York, NY: Pantheon Press, 1976.

Jarvis, De Forest Clinton. *Vermont Folk Medicine*. New York: Holt, 1958.

Kline, Monte L. and Strube, W.P.Jr. *Eat, Drink and Be Ready*. Fort Worth, TX: Harvest Press, Inc., 1977.

Kulvinskas, Viktoras. *Sprouts For The Love Of Every Body*. Wethersfield, CT: Omango D'Press, 1978.

Lambert, Edward C., M.D. *Modern Medical Mistakes*. Bloomington, IN: Indiana University Press, 1978.

Lesser, Michael, M.D. *Nutrition and Vitamin Therapy*. New York, NY: Random House Gross Press, Inc.

Mendelsohn, Robert S., M.D. *Confessions of a Medical Heretic*. Chicago, IL: Contemporary Books, 1979

Mendelsohn, Robert S., M.D. *How to Raise a Healthy Child in Spite of Your Doctor*. Chicago, IL: Contemporary Books, 1984.

Monroe, Esther. *Sprouts To Grow and Eat*. Brattleboro, VT: The Stephen Green Press, 1977.

Ott, John Nash. *Health and Light*. Greenwich, CT: Devin-Adair Publishers, Inc., 1974.

Pauling, Linus. *Vitamin C, the Common Cold, and the Flu*. San Francisco, CA: W.H. Freeman and Company, 1976.

Pfeiffer, Carl C. *Mental and Elemental Nutrients*. New Canaan, CT: Keats Publishing, Inc., 1975.

Philpott, William H., M.D. and Kalita, Dwight K., Ph.D. *Brain Allergy*. New Canaan, Ct: Keats Publishing, Inc., 1980.

Stedman, Thomas Lathrop. *Stedman's Medical Dictionary*. Baltimore: William and Wilkins, 1976.

Taylor, Renee. *Hunza Health Secrets for Long Life and Happiness*. Englewood Cliffs, NJ: Prentice Hall, Inc., 1971.

Williams, Roger J. *Nutrition Against Disease*. Marshfield, MA: Pitman Publishing, Inc., 1971.

Zack, Maura (Jinny) and Currier, Wilbur D., M.D. *Sugar Isn't Always Sweet*. Brea, CA: Uplift Books, 1983.

Index

A

Abcesses, 23–24
Abrahamson, E. M., 16
Acne, 24–25
Addison's disease, 17, 203–04
Aging, 25–27
AIDS (Acquired Immune
    Deficiency Syndrome),
    27–29 (*See also* Immune
    system)
Airola, Paavo, 83, 157
Alcoholism, 29–31
Allergies, 17, 24, *31–33*, 36–37,
    105–06, 170–71, 191–92
    (*See also* Kinesiology
    Testing)
Alternate therapists, 15, 18
Aluminum poisoning, 127
Alzheimer's Disease, 33–35
American Medical Association
    (AMA), 15
Anemia, 35–36
Anorexia, 36
*Appendix for Physicians in
    Brain Allergy,* 112
Arthritis, 36–37, 175–76, 188
    (*See also* Joint problems)
Artificial sweetners (*See*
    Sweetners, artificial)
Aslan, Dr. Ana, 26
Aspartame [NutraSweet] (*See*
    Sweetners, artificial)
Asthma, 17, 37
Astronauts, exercises of, 235–36
Athlete's foot, 37–38
Autism, 38

B

Bad breath (*See* Halitosis)
Balance, problems of, 39
Bandwagon to Health, 102, 157,
    207
Bedsores, 39
Bed-wetting, 39–40
Bee sting, 40
Behavior problems, 41–43
Be Your Own Doctor, 205, 222
Bible, references to and from, 13,
    20, 79, 89, 150, 205
Bland, Dr. Jeffrey, 48
Blood pressure, 17, 18, 56, 190
Body, Mind and Sugar, 16
Body pH Chart, 226–28
Bone Problems, 43–44
Bragg, Charles, 197
Bragg, Paul, 83
Brain Allergy, 86
Bronchitis, 44–46
Bruises, spontaneous, 46
Bunion, 46–47
Burns, 47
Bursitis, 47–48

C

Cadmium poisoning, 127
Caffeine, 225
Calories, understanding, 186–87,
    200
Calvin, Dr. Melvin, 221
Cancer, 48–50, 203–10 (*See also*
    Radiation damage)
Cancer Control Journal, 121

Cancer Control Society, 146
Candida Albicans, 29, 50–52
Canker sores, 52
Cataracts, 52–53
Cathcart, Dr. Richard, 48
Chelation, 53–54
Chemicals, 41–42, 127–28, 185,
     225 (*See also* Food
     additives and irradiation)
Chernobyl, 143
Chlorine, 54–55
Chlorophyll Green Drinks,
     223–24
Cholesterol problems, 17–18,
     55–56
Chronic Prostatitis, 139
Class, in weight control (*See*
     Weight control)
Claustrophobia, 56
Cold extremities, 56
Colds, 56–58
Cold sores (*See* Herpes,
     simplex)
Colic, 58–59
Colitis, 59–60
Conjunctivitis, 60
Constipation, 61–63
Cracked lips, 63

D

Dandruff, 64
Davis, Adelle, 17, 58
Deadly Don'ts, 224–25
Delirium tremens, 64
Depression, 33
DeSilva, Dr., 164–65
Diabetes, 64–65
Diagnostic test (*See* Hair
     analysis)
Diamond, Dr. John, 106, 138, 227
Diaper rash, 65–66
Diarrhea, 66–67, 155–56
Diets, 168, 177, 180–81, 187,
     213–16, 231 (*See also*
     Weight control)

Digestive system, 20
Directory of Products, Sources
     and Services, 237–39
Dizziness, 67–68
Doctors, nutrition oriented (*See*
     Alternate therapists)
Dorman, Dr. Purman, 75
Dreams, 68
Dribbling, of urine, 158
Drug allergy, 68–69
Dry mouth, 69
Dunn, Dr. Paul, 102
Dyslexia (*See* Autism)

E

Ear problems, 70–71
Economic food, 149, 214
Edema, 71–72
Edmonds, Alan, 114
Elizabeth's personal experiences
     cancer, triumphing over,
     203–10
     fasting, 79–83
     with penumonia, 136–37
Ellis, Dr. William A., 64, 227
Elton's personal experiences,
     210–12
Emotional disturbances (*See*
     Autism)
Emphysema, 72–73
*Encyclopedia of Common
     Disease, The*, 132
Energy problems, 73
Energy value of foods, 217–19,
     220
Enuresis (*See* Bed-wetting)
Environmental Protection
     Agency, 115
Epilepsy, 73–74
Equivalents (*See* Measurement/
     Equivalent Tables)
Esselbacher, Dr. Kurt, 114
Exercise, 74–75, 77, 94, 126,
     235–236
Exhaustion (*See* Energy

problems)
Eyes, 75–78, 188–95

F

Facial signs of health problems,
      78, 170–71, 174
Fasting, 78–84, 197, 208–09
Fasting, 83
Fatigue (*See* Energy problems)
Federal Department of
      Agriculture, 152
Fever, 84
Fever blisters, 84–85
Fingernail problems, 85–86,
      171–72
Flatulence, 86
Fluorescent lights, problems
      from, 87–88
Fluoride, 54–55
Folic acid deficiency, 88
Food additives, 88–89
Food and Drug Administration
      (FDA), 19, 88, 114, 115,
      118, 152
Foods with high, medium and
      low energy values, 217–19,
      220
Foot problems, 89
Frederick, Carlton, 16

G

Gallstones, 89–90
Gangrene, 90
Gas (*See* Flatulence)
Georgians, 22
Gerovital H3, 26
Glasses, colored or tinted, 77–78
Glaucoma, 90, 210–12
God, 13, 15, 20, 25, 28, 44, 50, 58,
      79, 83, 89, 98, 117, 123,
      130, 135, 136–37, 157,
      188, 199, 204, 205, 209,
      210

Goiter, 90
Goodheart, Dr. George, 138, 227
Gout, 91–92 (*See also* Joint
      (Problems)
Gray, Max; stories, 102–04,
      121–22
Growth problems (*See* Zinc
      deficiency)

H

Hair analysis, 92, 181–82,
      189–90
Hair problems, 92–93
Halitosis, 93
Harper, Dr. Harold; test, 209
Harvard Medical School, 114
Hay Fever, 93–94
Headache, 94–95
Health and Light, 87
Health food stores, merits of,
      216–17
Healthier Children/Happier
      Futures, 66
Health Institute of San Diego, 65
Hearing problems (*See* Ear
      problems)
Heart problems, 95–96
Hemorrhoids, 96–97
Hernia, 97–98
Herpes
      genital, 98
      simplex, 99
      zoster, 99–100
HGH, 169
Hiatial hernia (*See* Hernia)
High blood pressure, 184–85
      (*See* Hypertension)
Hippocrates, 65, 105
Hoffer, A., 30
Hormones, 168, 169
How to Get Well, 83
Hunzakuts, 21, 25
Hydrochloric acid deficiency,
      101

Hyperactivity, 101–04
Hypertension, 104–05
Hypochlorhydria, 106
Hypoglycemia, 16–17, 34–35,
    105–06, 232–34

I

Immune system, 106–07
Indigestion (*See* Stomach
    problems)
Infections, treatment for, 107
Infertility, 108–09
Insect stings, bites and poisons,
    40, 109–10
Insomnia, 110–11
Intestines, small; problems of,
    111–13
Ion Effect, The, 114
Ionization imbalance, 113–14
Irradiation, 114–15

J

Jarvis, Dr., 76
Jaws, underdevelopment of, 116
Joint problems, 116–17
Junk foods, 117–18
Juvenile delinquency, 119

K

Kidney problems, 119–20, 170
Kinesiology testing
    for adults, 227–32
    for children, 232
Klenner, Dr. Frederick T., 65,
    71, 90, 109, 210
Knutson, Dr. Richard A., 47

L

Large intestine (*See* Colon)
Lead poisoning, 126
Lethargy (*See* Energy problems)

Leukemia, 121–22
Lip Blisters (*See* Fever blisters)
Lips, cracked, 63
Live cell therapy, 26, 35, 107
Liver troubles, 122–23
Low blood sugar (*See*
    Hypoglycemia)
Low Blood Sugar and You, 16

M

Malabsorption, 123
Massachusetts Institute of
    Technology, 152
Mastication, need for, 124
Measurement/Equivalent
    Tables, 236
Meat, as an unhealthful food,
    20–21, 176–77, 200,
    213–15
Medical underground (*See*
    Alternate therapists)
Memory loss, 124–25
Mendelsohn, Dr. Robert, 19, 71,
    150
Meniere's disease (*See*
    Dizziness)
Menstruation, 125–26
*Mental and Elemental
    Nutrients,* 38
Mental problems (*See* Autism)
Mercury poisoning, 127
Metal Poisoning, 126–28
Milk, 114–15, 117, 118
Mineral deficiencies, 128,
    182–83
Mooreburn, Dr. Elsie, 181, 184
Motion sickness, 128
Mouth problems, 129
Multiple sclerosis, 129–30
Munger, Dr., 171
Muscle spasms, stiffness,
    soreness, 130–31, 183–84
Muscle strength test (*See*
    Kinesiology Testing)

N

Natural Health Magazine of Australia, 28
Natural Health Society of Australia, 215
Nausea (*See* Motion sickness)
Nervousness, 169
Neuralgia, 131–32
Neuritis, 131–32
Niehans, Dr., 26
Night blindness, 132–33
Nightmares (*See* Dreams)
Nolfi, Dr. Christine, 205
Numbness of extremities, 133
Nutrition Against Disease, 29
Nutrition Almanac, The, 169
Nutritional News, 18

O

Obesity (*See* Weight control)
Oils, fats, 177, 224
Organically grown food, 216
Osler, Sir William, 95
Osmond, H., 30
Osteoporosis (*See* Bone problems)
Ott, Dr. John N., 87
Overweight (*See* Weight control)
Oxygen problems (*See* Emphysema)

P

Pain, 133–34
Palsy (*See* Parkinson's disease)
Pancreatitis, 134–35
Pardridge, Dr. William, 152
Parkinson's disease, 135, 196–97
Pauling, Dr. Linus, 48, 56
Peget, A. V., 16
Pfeiffer, Carl C., Ph.D., M.D., 38
pH, in the body, 57, 73, 84, 120, 132, **225–27**

Philpott, Dr. William, 86, 112
Physician's Desk Reference, 68, 196
Physicians, orthodox, 19
Pigmentation problems (*See* Vitiligo)
Piles (*See* Hemorrhoids)
Pliny, 159
Pneumonia, 135–37
Poison Ivy, Poison Oak, 138
Post nasal drip, 138–39
Prescription drugs (*See* Drug allergy)
Prevention magazine, 132
Processed foods, 18
Produce, need for washing, 192
Professionals, nutrition oriented (*See* Alternate therapists)
Prostaglandin, 168
Prostate problems, 139
Psoriasis, 139–40
Pyorrhea, 140–41

R

Radiation, 19, 69, 141–43, 222
Randolph, Dr. Theron, 79, 80
Raw foods, 48–49, 72, 98, 129–30, 149–50, 206–07
Raynaud's syndrome, 143–44
Recipes for Chlorophyll Green Drinks, 223–24
Respiratory diseases (*See* Asthma, Bronchitis, Emphysema, Smoking)
Respiratory infections (*See* Colds)
Retinosa Pigmentosa, 144–45
Rodaquin, 26–27, 35
Rupture (*See* Hernia)

S

Scars, help for, 142–43
Science Magazine, 52
Shefrin, Dr., 97

Shingles (*See* Herpes, Zoster)

Silver, Dr. Lloyd H., 11, 183

Sinus irrigation directions,
   45–46

Sjorgren's syndrome (*See* Dry
   mouth)

Skin cancers, 145–46

Small Intestine (*See* Intestine,
   small; problems of)

Smoking, snuff and tobacco
   chewing, 146–47

Somatotropin, 168

Sore throat (*See* Colds)

Soyka, Fred, 114

Sprains, strains, torn ligaments,
   147–48

Sprouts, 149, 157, 194

Stedman's Medical Dictionary,
   97, 131, 135

Stress; Physical, mental,
   emotional, 149–50

Strontium 90 contamination,
   127, 143

Sudden infant death syndrome,
   150

Sugar
   addiction to, 174
   as a cure for wounds, 107
   avoidance of, 17, 224
   causes behavior problems, 41,
      102, 119
   natural replacements for,
      185–86
   robs body of nutrients, 18

Sugar Blues, 175, 178

Supplements, pros and cons of,
   219–20

Surgery, 19, 150–52

Sweetners, artificial, 118, 152,
   185

T

Taylor, Renee, 21

Teeth, humankinds reason for,
   20

Thermal Burns (*See* Burns)

Thyroid, 170 (*See also* Goiter)

Tic Douloreaux, 153

Tobacco addiction (*See*
   Smoking)

Tongue, as an indicator of ill
   health, 172–73

Tonsillitis, 153–54

Tooth Problems, 154–55

Torn ligaments (*See* Sprains,
   Strains)

*Treatment of Schizophrenia
   Nicotinin Acid or
   Nicotinomide*, 30

Turista, 155–56

U

Ulcerated fungus (*See* Candida
   Albicans)

Ulcers, stomach and duodenal,
   157

UNcook Book, The, 11, 39, 157,
   207

Urine problems, 158

V

Vaginitis, 158–59

Varicose veins, 159

Vegetarianism, 20–22, 213–16

Vermont Folk Medicine, 76

Vertigo (*See* Dizziness)

Vietti, Dr., 90

Virno, Dr., 90

*Vitamin C and the Common
   Cold*, 56

Vitiligo, 159–60

W

Walker, Sidney, M.D.M., 102

Warts, 160–61

Water blisters (*See* Herpes,
   simplex)

Weight control, 161–63,

167-201
Wheat grass, beauties of, 221-24
Whitehead, 163
Wigmore, Ann, 205, 222
Williams, Dr. Roger, 29
Worms, 163-65
Wound infection dressing, 47
Wurtman, Dr. Richard, 152

X

Xerostomic (*See* dry mouth)

X-ray, 19 (*See also* Radiation
   damage)

Y

Your Body Doesn't Lie, 106, 138

Z

Zinc deficiency, 165-66
Zion International Hospital, 79

HELP A FRIEND OR LOVED ONE TO BETTER HEALTH

There's nothing like having you own personal copy of *The UNmedical Book!* Then you can refer to it whenever the need arises. To order your copy or one for a friend, simply complete the form below and include your check or money order.

MORE IMPORTANT BOOKS BY THE BAKERS...

The UNcook Book offers raw food adventures to a new health high. It's a unique and practical cookbook chock-full of delicious recipes. There are also chapters on sprouting, traveling, eating out, how to combine foods for good digestion, etc. Now *in its fourth printing,* this book has led thousands of people back to health. Only $5.95

Bandwagon to Health is a comprehensive handbook which takes readers through an easy Seven Phase Program leading from the typical American conventional diet to a healthful, all-natural way of eating. It contains a rich appendix with vitamin and mineral data and food composition charts. $6.95

ORDER BLANK

The UNmedical Book @ $8.95   quantity _____ $_____
The UNcook Book   @ $5.95   quantity _____ $_____
Bandwagon to Health @ $6.95   quantity _____ $_____

Subtotal $_____
Shipping ($2 per book) $_____
Tax (CO residents 3%) $_____

TOTAL $_____

Note: Canadian orders must be accompanied by a U.S. postal money order. Allow 30-45 days for delivery.

Name _____
Address _____Phone( ) _____
City/State/Zip _____

Make your check or money order payable to:
COMMUNICATION CREATIVITY, Box 213, Saguache, CO 81149

BULK ORDERS INVITED—call (303) 589-8223 or (303) 589-5995